Caffeine in Food and Dietary Supplements

Examining Safety

WORKSHOP SUMMARY

Leslie Pray, Ann L. Yaktine, and Diana Pankevich, *Rapporteurs*

Planning Committee for a Workshop on Potential Health Hazards Associated with Consumption of Caffeine in Food and Dietary Supplements

Food and Nutrition Board

Board on Health Sciences Policy

INSTITUTE OF MEDICINE
OF THE NATIONAL ACADEMIES

THE NATIONAL ACADEMIES PRESS
Washington, D.C.
www.nap.edu

THE NATIONAL ACADEMIES PRESS • 500 Fifth Street, NW • Washington, DC 20001

NOTICE: The workshop that is the subject of this workshop summary was approved by the Governing Board of the National Research Council, whose members are drawn from the councils of the National Academy of Sciences, the National Academy of Engineering, and the Institute of Medicine.

This activity was supported by Contract/Grant No. HHSF223200810020I between the National Academy of Sciences and the Department of Health and Human Services, Food and Drug Administration. The views presented in this publication do not necessarily reflect the views of the organizations or agencies that provided support for the activity.

International Standard Book Number-13: 978-0-309-29749-3
International Standard Book Number-10: 0-309-29749-4

Additional copies of this workshop summary are available for sale from the National Academies Press, 500 Fifth Street, NW, Keck 360, Washington, DC 20001; (800) 624-6242 or (202) 334-3313; http://www.nap.edu.

For more information about the Institute of Medicine, visit the IOM home page at **www.iom.edu.**

Printed in the United States of America

The serpent has been a symbol of long life, healing, and knowledge among almost all cultures and religions since the beginning of recorded history. The serpent adopted as a logotype by the Institute of Medicine is a relief carving from ancient Greece, now held by the Staatliche Museen in Berlin.

Suggested citation: IOM (Institute of Medicine). 2014. *Caffeine in food and dietary supplements: Examining safety: Workshop summary.* Washington, DC: The National Academies Press.

"Knowing is not enough; we must apply.
Willing is not enough; we must do."
—Goethe

INSTITUTE OF MEDICINE
OF THE NATIONAL ACADEMIES

Advising the Nation. Improving Health.

THE NATIONAL ACADEMIES

Advisers to the Nation on Science, Engineering, and Medicine

The **National Academy of Sciences** is a private, nonprofit, self-perpetuating society of distinguished scholars engaged in scientific and engineering research, dedicated to the furtherance of science and technology and to their use for the general welfare. Upon the authority of the charter granted to it by the Congress in 1863, the Academy has a mandate that requires it to advise the federal government on scientific and technical matters. Dr. Ralph J. Cicerone is president of the National Academy of Sciences.

The **National Academy of Engineering** was established in 1964, under the charter of the National Academy of Sciences, as a parallel organization of outstanding engineers. It is autonomous in its administration and in the selection of its members, sharing with the National Academy of Sciences the responsibility for advising the federal government. The National Academy of Engineering also sponsors engineering programs aimed at meeting national needs, encourages education and research, and recognizes the superior achievements of engineers. Dr. C. D. Mote, Jr., is president of the National Academy of Engineering.

The **Institute of Medicine** was established in 1970 by the National Academy of Sciences to secure the services of eminent members of appropriate professions in the examination of policy matters pertaining to the health of the public. The Institute acts under the responsibility given to the National Academy of Sciences by its congressional charter to be an adviser to the federal government and, upon its own initiative, to identify issues of medical care, research, and education. Dr. Harvey V. Fineberg is president of the Institute of Medicine.

The **National Research Council** was organized by the National Academy of Sciences in 1916 to associate the broad community of science and technology with the Academy's purposes of furthering knowledge and advising the federal government. Functioning in accordance with general policies determined by the Academy, the Council has become the principal operating agency of both the National Academy of Sciences and the National Academy of Engineering in providing services to the government, the public, and the scientific and engineering communities. The Council is administered jointly by both Academies and the Institute of Medicine. Dr. Ralph J. Cicerone and Dr. C. D. Mote, Jr., are chair and vice chair, respectively, of the National Research Council.

www.national-academies.org

PLANNING COMMITTEE FOR A WORKSHOP ON POTENTIAL HEALTH HAZARDS ASSOCIATED WITH CONSUMPTION OF CAFFEINE IN FOOD AND DIETARY SUPPLEMENTS[1]

LYNN R. GOLDMAN (*Chair*), Dean, School of Public Health and Health Sciences George Washington University, Washington, DC
JAMES R. COUGHLIN, President, Coughlin & Associates, San Diego, CA
STEPHEN R. DANIELS, Professor and Chair, Department of Pediatrics, University of Colorado, Aurora
THOMAS J. GOULD, Professor of Psychology, Department of Psychology, Director of the Neuroscience Program, Temple University, Philadelphia, PA
CARL L. KEEN, Professor and Chair, Department of Nutrition, University of California, Davis
STEVEN E. LIPSHULTZ, Professor and Chairman of Pediatrics and Endowed Chair in Pediatric Cardiology, Children's Hospital of the University of Miami, FL
THERESA ANN NICKLAS, Professor, Department of Pediatrics, Children's Nutrition Research Center, Baylor College of Medicine, Houston, TX
BARBARA J. PETERSEN, Principal Scientist, Exponent, Inc., Washington, DC
JOSEPH V. RODRICKS, Principal, Environ International Corp., Arlington, VA

IOM Staff

ANN L. YAKTINE, Study Director
DIANA PANKEVICH, Senior Program Officer
JANET MULLIGAN, Research Associate
FAYE HILLMAN, Financial Associate
GERALDINE KENNEDO, Administrative Assistant
ANN L. YAKTINE, Interim Director, Food and Nutrition Board
ANDREW M. POPE, Director, Board on Health Sciences Policy

---

[1]Institute of Medicine planning committees are solely responsible for organizing the workshop, identifying topics, and choosing speakers. The responsibility for the published workshop summary rests with the workshop rapporteurs and the institution.

Reviewers

This workshop summary has been reviewed in draft form by individuals chosen for their diverse perspectives and technical expertise, in accordance with procedures approved by the National Research Council's Report Review Committee. The purpose of this independent review is to provide candid and critical comments that will assist the institution in making its published workshop summary as sound as possible and to ensure that the workshop summary meets institutional standards for objectivity, evidence, and responsiveness to the study charge. The review comments and draft manuscript remain confidential to protect the integrity of the process. We wish to thank the following individuals for their review of this workshop summary:

ANNE BARNHILL, Perelman School of Medicine at the University of Pennsylvania
CINDY D. DAVIS, National Institutes of Health
JOHANNA T. DWYER, Tufts University Medical Center
CARL L. KEEN, University of California, Davis
NANCY S. WELLMAN, Florida International University

Although the reviewers listed above have provided many constructive comments and suggestions, they did not see the final draft of the workshop summary before its release. The review of this workshop summary was overseen by **EILEEN T. KENNEDY,** Tufts University. Appointed by the Institute of Medicine, she was responsible for making certain that an independent examination of this workshop summary was carried out in accordance with institutional procedures and that all review comments were carefully considered. Responsibility for the final content of this workshop summary rests entirely with the rapporteurs and the institution.

Contents

Boxes, Figures, and Tables

BOXES

FIGURES

TABLES

Abbreviations and Acronyms

ADHD	attention deficit hyperactivity disorder
CDC	U.S. Centers for Disease Control and Prevention
COMT	catechol-O-methyltransferase
CRN	Council for Responsible Nutrition
DAWN	Drug Abuse Warning Network
DSM	*Diagnostic and Statistical Manual*
ECF	endothelial cell function
EFSA	European Food Safety Authority
FDA	U.S. Food and Drug Administration
GABA	gamma-aminobutyric acid
GRAS	generally recognized as safe
ILSI	International Life Sciences Institute
IOM	Institute of Medicine
MSN	medium spiny neuron
NHANES	National Health and Nutrition Examination Survey
NOAEL	no-observed-adverse-effect level
NPDS	National Poison Data System
PVC	premature ventricular complex

QT	Q-T wave
RACC	reference amount customarily consumed
SHADE-ONE	**S**tudy of **H**eart Effects from **A**dults **D**rinking **E**nergy Beverages: **On E**ndothelial Function

1

Introduction[1]

BACKGROUND AND WORKSHOP OBJECTIVES

Caffeine, a central nervous system stimulant, is arguably the most frequently ingested pharmacologically active substance in the world. Occurring naturally in more than 60 plants, including coffee beans, tea leaves, cola nuts, and cocoa pods, caffeine has been part of innumerable cultures for centuries. But the caffeine-in-food landscape is changing. From waffles to sunflower seeds, jelly beans to syrup, and even bottled water, the array of new caffeine-containing energy products, including energy drinks and supplements entering the marketplace, is, in the words of U.S. Food and Drug Administration (FDA) commissioner Margaret Hamburg, "truly mind boggling." Years of scientific research have shown that moderate consumption by healthy adults of products containing naturally occurring caffeine is not associated with adverse health effects. But the changing caffeine landscape raises concerns about safety and whether any of these new products might be targeting populations not normally associated with caffeine consumption, namely, children and adolescents, and whether caffeine poses a greater health risk to those populations than it does to healthy adults.

At the request of the FDA, on August 5–6, 2013, the Institute of Medicine (IOM) convened a workshop in Washington, DC, to review the

[1]The planning committee's role was limited to planning the workshop, and the workshop summary has been prepared by the workshop rapporteurs as a factual summary of what occurred at the workshop. Statements, recommendations, and opinions expressed are those of individual presenters and participants and are not necessarily endorsed or verified by the Institute of Medicine, and they should not be construed as reflecting any group consensus.

available science on safe levels of caffeine consumption in foods, beverages, and dietary supplements and to identify data gaps. See Box 1-1 for a detailed list of specific workshop objectives. Workshop participants included scientists with expertise in food safety, nutrition, pharmacology, psychology, toxicology, and related disciplines; medical professionals with pediatric and adult patient experience in cardiology, neurology, and psychiatry; public health professionals; food industry representatives; regulatory experts; and consumer advocates.

The information presented in this workshop summary reflects only what was spoken or visually presented (on slides) during the workshop. Although this workshop summary covers a range of subject matter, it should not be construed as a comprehensive review of the subject matter. Nor should any of the information, opinions, or conclusions expressed here be construed as reflecting consensus on the part of the IOM, the Food and Nutrition Board, the Board on Health Sciences Policy, the workshop planning committee, or any group. The purpose of the workshop was to engage in a dialogue about the safety of caffeine in food and dietary supplements, including, but not limited to, caffeinated beverage products, and to identify data gaps, not to reach consensus on any issue or to make recommendations. All the opinions, interpretations, and suggestions for future research summarized in this document reflect the opinions of individual workshop participants.

Equally important, although much of the workshop discussion revolved around the science of the safety of caffeine in energy drink beverages, the intended scope of the workshop discussion extended across all foods and beverages, as well as dietary supplements, and included coffee, tea, carbonated soft drinks, and numerous other types of products. Also, as the planning committee chair Lynn Goldman emphasized in her welcoming remarks, the workshop was intended to cover only the assessment of potential health risks associated with caffeine exposure (i.e., risk assessment), not the management of those risks (i.e., risk management).

ABOUT THIS REPORT

The organization of this report roughly parallels the workshop objectives and organization of the workshop itself. The major overarching themes of the workshop, reflected in the chapter summaries, are shown

BOX 1-1
Workshop Objectives

- Evaluate the epidemiological, toxicological, clinical, and other relevant literature to describe important health hazards associated with caffeine consumption.
- Delineate vulnerable populations who may be at risk from caffeine exposure. Describe caffeine exposure and the risk of cardiovascular and other health effects on vulnerable populations, including additive effects with other ingredients and effects related to preexisting conditions.
- Explore safe caffeine exposure levels for general and vulnerable populations. Identify data gaps on caffeine stimulant effects, including but not limited to cardiovascular, central nervous system, or other health outcomes.

in Box 1-2. This first introductory chapter contains a summary of introductory remarks made by Margaret A. Hamburg, commissioner of the FDA, and Michael R. Taylor, deputy commissioner for foods and veterinary medicine at the FDA, and it includes a list of major overarching themes of the workshop discussion, compiled by the rapporteurs.

Chapter 2 summarizes the workshop presentations and discussion on methods being used to assess levels of caffeine exposure in the U.S. general population. Chapter 3 summarizes the presentations and discussion of the different types of surveillance in place for identifying safety signals related to caffeine. Although the challenge of gaining a better scientific understanding of potentially vulnerable populations was addressed throughout the workshop in different contexts, Chapter 4 summarizes the one panel that focused specifically on vulnerable populations. Chapter 5 summarizes the presentations and discussion of the current state of the science on the risk of cardiovascular disease associated with caffeine exposure—in both general and vulnerable populations. Chapter 6 summarizes the several panels dedicated to exploring the effects of caffeine exposure on the central nervous system and behavior, again in both general and vulnerable populations. Chapter 7 summarizes the workshop presentations and discussion on the interactions between caffeine and other ingredients in caffeine-containing foods and dietary supplements. At the end of Day 1, workshop participants were invited to comment on any issue, with three minutes provided per participant. Chapter 8 summarizes those remarks. Finally, Chapter 9 summarizes the final session of the day, a panel on data gaps and ways to fill those gaps.

THE PAST, PRESENT, AND FUTURE OF CAFFEINE REGULATION IN THE UNITED STATES

Introductory Remarks Given by Margaret A. Hamburg, M.D., Commissioner of the FDA, and Michael R. Taylor, J.D., Deputy Commissioner for Foods and Veterinary Medicine at the FDA

Caffeine in cola-type beverages has been listed as generally recognized as safe (GRAS) since 1959 (i.e., in cola up to 200 parts per million, or about 70 mg in a 12-ounce serving, in accordance with good manufacturing practices). Nevertheless, even early on, according to FDA commissioner Margaret Hamburg, there were concerns about the effects of caffeine consumption beyond moderate levels and in children, pregnant women, and other potentially vulnerable populations.[2] In a 1978 report, the Select Committee on GRAS Substances raised questions about whether the chronic consumption of caffeine in cola-type beverages by children during a period of brain growth and development might affect behavior (FDA, 1989). The evidence was inconclusive. More recently, in response to the influx of caffeinated alcoholic beverages into the marketplace, in 2010 the FDA sent four warning letters to manufacturers of those beverages. The beverages were subsequently removed from the

BOX 1-2
Major Overarching Themes of Workshop Discussion

- Although the health effects of caffeine have a long history of scientific study, caffeine is being marketed to consumers in novel products and in new ways, raising new questions about caffeine intake and the health consequences of caffeine exposure.
- Many unanswered questions exist about actual exposure levels, especially among children and adolescents, who have historically not consumed much caffeine but are increasingly consuming it in the form of caffeinated energy drinks and other food products, including questions about physiologic responses to caffeine in naïve users.

[2]For the purposes of this discussion, moderate intake of caffeine for the healthy adult population is defined as a dose level up to 400 mg/day (equivalent to 6 mg/kg body weight/day in a 65-kg person). Excessive intake of caffeine is considered to be greater than 500–600 mg/day (8.3–10 mg/kg) (4–7 cups of coffee or 7–9 cups of tea). Caffeine intake that is greater than 400 mg/day (6.7 mg/kg) "may increase the risk of detrusor instability (unstable bladder) development in women" (Nawrot et al., 2003).

BOX 1-2 Continued

- Scientific evidence on cardiovascular effects associated with caffeine exposure is varied and incomplete. Scientists have examined several different end points, from arrhythmia to vasodilation, with mixed results. There are many unanswered questions about individual and population variability (e.g., some individuals may be genetically susceptible to cardiovascular effects associated with caffeine intake; some populations, particularly children and adolescents, may be more vulnerable than others), as well as the nature of the caffeine exposure (e.g., caffeine consumed in combination with one set of ingredients may have very different cardiovascular effects than caffeine consumed in combination with another set of ingredients).
- As with cardiovascular effects, scientists have examined various central nervous system and behavioral effects of caffeine exposure. The evidence raises several questions about the safety of exposure in children and adolescents in particular. Little is known about the interactions between caffeine and other ingredients in caffeine-containing foods and dietary supplements and whether and how those interactions alter the health effects of caffeine exposure.
- While most of the discussion of vulnerable populations focused on children, adolescents, and pregnant women, some participants expressed concern that not enough scientific evidence has been collected to clearly identify vulnerability. Participants identified children with underlying heart medical conditions as a separate potentially vulnerable population and identified individuals with certain genetic predispositions as another.
- There was some controversy over the urgency of the sudden cardiac death safety signal being observed in adolescents, with some workshop participants expressing concern that the signal was being sensationalized. Others emphasized that although not all clinicians may be seeing the signal, clearly some are, not just in the United States, but globally. Several calls were put forth to advance the discussion beyond a debate over whether a safety signal exists and to consider ways that the signal can be scientifically investigated. Suggestions were put forth to improve and systematize the collection of exposure and both short-term and long-term health outcome data by popularizing the National Poison Control Center database, developing a national registry, or conducting longitudinal cohort studies.

market. As Hamburg explained, the FDA had not approved the use of caffeine in alcoholic beverages at any level and was concerned about their safety in light of published peer-reviewed studies suggesting that the consumption of beverages with added caffeine and alcohol is associated with risk behaviors. Caffeine appears to mask some of the sensory cues individuals might otherwise rely on to determine their level of intoxication.

Hamburg noted that although caffeinated beverages containing alcohol are no longer on U.S. shelves, the energy drink marketplace has continued to expand and is, today, a multi-billion-dollar business. The products come in a range of sizes and are marketed as either conventional beverages or dietary supplements. Several contain other compounds that interact with the added caffeine or add yet another effect. Many of these products, just as with other products with added caffeine, appeal especially or even particularly to a young audience.

Hamburg identified three primary points she hoped workshop participants would focus on during the course of the next day and a half. First, she asked workshop participants to examine the health risks associated with the use of caffeine beyond moderate levels and for specific populations. Some studies have suggested that heavier consumption or habitual use of caffeine increases these risks, particularly for vulnerable populations, such as among pregnant women and children. For example, the literature suggests that there may be reproductive effects, such as reduced fertility and decreased birth weight, even at lower intake levels (Fenster et al., 1991; Klebanoff et al., 1999). In addition, there is limited evidence of anxiety in children at low doses (Bernstein et al., 1994). By examining and evaluating the epidemiological, toxicological, clinical, and other literature, workshop participants will help the FDA to gain a better and more complete understanding of health risks for these various populations of concern.

Second, Hamburg requested that workshop participants focus on issues surrounding the marketplace for these products, including expanded availability of caffeine and conditions under which these products are used. She noted that the American Academy of Pediatrics, as well as the report *Nutrition Standards for Foods in Schools* (IOM, 2007), have expressed concern about making caffeine more readily accessible and attractive to children and adolescents. The FDA needs to know what the research suggests about caffeine exposure, particularly the additive effects and the conditions under which it is used, including in energy drinks and similar sources, and whether the FDA should be more closely monitoring and regulating these products, especially in vulnerable populations.

Third, the FDA intends to be as transparent as possible in its investigation and study of this area and these kinds of products. To that end, it has worked cooperatively with the food and beverage industries, who have shared their expertise and experience, and has reached out to public health and medical specialty groups as well as to consumers and consumer advocates. The agency has also conducted preliminary analyses of available adverse-event databases. But, Hamburg said, now is the time to delve as deeply as possible and draw on all the expertise available.

Hamburg remarked that she and her FDA colleagues are encouraged by how some in the industry have responded to concerns about the risk that children could be overexposed to caffeine, as demonstrated by Wrigley's recent announcement not to market a chewing gum that it had developed with caffeine. Such voluntary restraint is helpful at this time when the FDA is still searching for information and considering how better to define the regulatory boundaries around caffeine. Hamburg said the agency looks forward to continuing to work with the different parts of industry. But despite the laudable restraint that the FDA has seen in some instances, Hamburg observed that it knows that some companies have been adding caffeine to their products on the basis of their opinion that such use is GRAS, and they have done so without engaging the FDA. As a result, those companies are raising numerous questions about the scope and rigor of their safety analyses. That approach threatens to implicate the credibility of the industry as a whole and potentially undermine the FDA's carefully balanced regulatory oversight, which is designed to allow innovation while ensuring safety and public confidence.

A goal for this workshop was to allow the FDA to take a close and thorough look at what is happening in the marketplace, how industry is proceeding, and what actions may be necessary. Hamburg opined that the workshop was occurring at a critical time and, as such, offered a critical opportunity to evaluate the data and to reach some informed conclusions. She said, "I really do believe that the deliberations that you will be undertaking over the next 2 days, the discussions that you will be having, the data presented, [and] the issues raised will all help to guide us as we consider the right steps forward to protect public health."

On the second day of the workshop, Mike Taylor, FDA Deputy Commissioner for Foods and Veterinary Medicine, emphasized the need to "get the science right" in determining whether there are safety concerns regarding the new uses of caffeine that warrant steps by the FDA. He elaborated on how the issues being addressed are not simple. Caffeine is not an ordinary food additive. It is a central nervous system stimulant, a drug with multiple effects in the human body. It is different from virtually everything else that the FDA regulates as added ingredients in food because consumers seek it out for its pharmacologic effect. Taylor noted, as Hamburg had, that caffeine had been a part of human history for centuries, with the traditional uses of caffeine being apparently safe for healthy adults. Today, however, caffeine is available in a much wider variety of food products, as well as dietary supplement products, and is being consumed in a wider range of use conditions.

Taylor underscored the importance of specifically addressing the new forms of caffeine and caffeine consumption scenarios that are attractive or accessible to children and adolescents. Do these new use conditions raise new safety questions? How do we assess the intake resulting from these new exposure scenarios created by the wider availability of caffeine and by the fact that caffeine is, again, a sought-after ingredient for people wishing to experience its physiological effects? Are there special measures needed to address and possibly protect vulnerable populations? Again, "getting the science right" is the first crucial step, Taylor said. This IOM workshop was intended to help the FDA to do that.

Further complicating the issue for the FDA is the fact that these questions must be addressed not in the abstract but in the context of the two regulatory frameworks provided by Congress to oversee ingredients in the food supply and in dietary supplements (see Box 1-3). The first regulatory framework, which addresses dietary supplement products, was established by the Dietary Supplement Health and Education Act in the 1990s. It is aimed at products designed to supplement the diet with ingredients that presumably provide beneficial effects to consumers. These products are permissible in the market unless there is significant or unreasonable risk of illness or injury under the labeled or ordinary conditions of use. For dietary ingredients that are not new, the burden is on the FDA to prove that the safety standard or risk standard has been exceeded.

The second regulatory framework, the 1958 food additive law (Food Additives Amendment to the Food, Drug and Cosmetic Act), addresses the safety of ingredients that are added to conventional foods to provide traditional food functions such as nutrition, flavor, and hydration. According to Taylor, it requires a higher standard of safety, that is, the "reasonable certainty of no harm" safety standard established by Congress for added ingredients in food. Under the food additive law, the burden is on industry to prove safety, and there is a prescribed pre-market approval process for food additives. The GRAS concept provides an alternative pathway to the marketplace, one that does not require FDA pre-market approval. The GRAS concept is an important feature of the framework. GRAS status determination must be based on the same quantity and quality of evidence required, as though the substance were being approved by the FDA as a food additive, that is, with a reasonable certainty of no harm. In addition, there must be general recognition that the safety standard has been met based on publicly available data and information.

BOX 1-3
Dietary Supplements

A "dietary supplement," as defined by Congress in the Dietary Supplement and Education Act of 1994, is a product taken by mouth that contains a "dietary ingredient" intended to supplement the diet. Such ingredients may include "vitamins, minerals, herbs or other botanicals, amino acids, and substances such as enzymes, organ tissues, glandulars, and metabolites." Dietary supplements can also be "extracts or concentrates, and may be found in many forms such as tablets, capsules, softgels, gelcaps, liquids, or powders." If a dietary supplement is in a bar, information on the label "must not represent the product as a conventional food or a sole item of a meal or diet."

SOURCE: U.S. Food and Drug Administration. Available at http://www.fda.gov/Food/DietarySupplements/QADietarySupplements/default.htm#what_is.

Despite differences between the two regulatory frameworks, both provide similar options potentially available to the FDA. Taylor underscored "potentially." He remarked that the FDA had not made any decisions (about caffeine being added to new products) and had no preconceived notions of what the right steps are. If the science justifies doing so, under either framework the FDA can potentially restrict levels of caffeine in products or conditions of use. The agency could also use labeling to inform consumers about the amount of caffeine in products or provide cautionary statements where appropriate.

Taylor stressed that, regardless of which framework the FDA decides to operate under, the science is still the same with respect to how caffeine affects the body and whether there are effects that should be addressed in vulnerable populations.

On behalf of the FDA, Taylor said, he appreciated the call put forth during the workshop by the Grocery Manufacturers Association to collaborate with the FDA on defining boundaries around the use of caffeine (see Chapter 8). He also expressed gratitude for the restraint that many food companies have been exercising as the FDA works on what Taylor described as an "extraordinarily complex scientific puzzle, regulatory puzzle, [and] public health puzzle."

REFERENCES

Bernstein, G. A., M. E. Carroll, R. D. Crosby, A. R. Perwien, F. S. Go, and N. L. Benowitz. 1994. Caffeine effects on learning, performance, and anxiety in normal school-age children. *Journal of the American Academy of Child and Adolescent Psychiatry* 33(3):407–415.

FDA (Food and Drug Administration). 1989. *Select Committee on GRAS Substances (SCOGS) report no. 89: Caffeine.* http://ww.accessdata.fda.gov/scripts/fcn/fcnDetailNavigation.cfm?rpt=scogsListing&id=42 (accessed January 13, 2014).

Fenster, L., B. Eskenazi, G. C. Windham, and S. H. Swan. 1991. Caffeine consumption during pregnancy and spontaneous abortion. *Epidemiology* 2:168–174.

IOM (Institute of Medicine). 2007. *Nutrition standards for foods in schools: Leading the way toward healthier youth.* Washington, DC: The National Academies Press.

Klebanoff, M. A., R. J. Levine, R. DerSimonian, J. D. Clemens, and D. G. Wilkins. 1999. Maternal serum paraxanthine, a caffeine metabolite, and the risk of spontaneous abortion. *New England Journal of Medicine* 341:1639–1644.

Nawrot, P., S. Jordan, J. Eastwood, J. Rotstein, A. Hugenholtz, and M. Feeley. 2003. Effects of caffeine on human health. *Food Additives and Contaminants* 20:1–30.

2

Intake and Exposure to Caffeine[1]

Given the large and growing number of different sources of caffeine, assessing the level of caffeine exposure is an important and complex first step toward understanding the safety of such exposure. In the Day 1, Session 1, panel, moderated by Barbara J. Petersen, Ph.D., M.P.H., of Exponent, panelists considered different methods being used to assess levels of caffeine exposure in the U.S. general population. Petersen emphasized that different methods yield different results and that the results presented here should not be interpreted as final answers. For her, a key question to consider is how people behave when a source of caffeine disappears or a new source appears and whether people substitute one source for another. This chapter summarizes the panelists' presentations and the discussion that followed. Key points made by each speaker are shown in Box 2-1.

CAFFEINE INTAKE FROM BEVERAGES IN THE UNITED STATES

Presented by Diane C. Mitchell, M.S., R.D., Pennsylvania State University

The International Life Sciences Institute (ILSI) has supported research on caffeine since 1983, resulting in several publications (e.g., Knight et al., 2004, 2006). Diane Mitchell presented ILSI's most recent

[1]The words "exposure" and "intake" were used interchangeably throughout the workshop.

caffeine study, which was conducted in collaboration with Kantar Worldpanel (Mitchell et al., 2013). The primary objective of the study was to estimate caffeine intakes in the United States from the consumption of caffeinated beverages using a current (2010–2011) population-based beverage survey. According to Mitchell, the study was conducted primarily because of the lack of comprehensive, current, and reliable population-based data on caffeine intakes. Most studies examining exposure to caffeine in the United States were surveys conducted more than a decade ago, including research sponsored by ILSI. The data provide a current perspective on patterns of beverage caffeine exposure in the United States in the total population as well as in demographic subgroups. They not only update past ILSI-sponsored research, but they also provide an opportunity to compare trends in beverage caffeine intakes between then and now.

BOX 2-1
Key Points Made by Individual Speakers

According to Diane Mitchell, most studies examining exposure to caffeine in the United States were conducted more than 10 years ago.

Mitchell described the methods and results of a recent study on caffeine intakes from beverages in the United States. The study, conducted by the International Life Sciences Institute, was the first population-based study of caffeine intakes from beverages in the United States in more than a decade. The survey included 7 days of online dietary records entered daily by each respondent. Data collection excluded children under 2 years of age. Data collected included type, brand, preparation, location, and amount of all beverages consumed. In sum, mean daily intake was 165 mg per day, compared to 120 mg per day in 1999. Most beverage caffeine intake in the United States comes from coffee and, to a lesser extent, tea and carbonated soft drinks, with energy drinks contributing very little. Energy drink consumption was not estimated in the 1999 survey. In Mitchell's opinion, the data do not support the notion that the introduction of additional caffeinated beverages into the marketplace has resulted in proportionately higher caffeine intakes by consumers.

Victor Fulgoni III described four approaches to analyzing caffeine intake data from the National Health and Nutrition Examination Survey (NHANES): usual intake, intake per consumption event, trends in intake over time, and trends in intake over time by food source. The data cover all foods and beverages, but not dietary supplements, with more than 90 percent of caffeine intake coming from beverages. Data were collected from one 24-hour in-person dietary recall, and for a subset of participants a second recall was conducted by phone. For trend data, Fulgoni used only the single in-person intake day. Survey participation was not limited by age. Data collected included all foods and beverages consumed. In sum, the data demonstrate stable intakes between 2001 and 2010. If anything, some age groups show slight decreases in caffeine intake. With respect to food sources, there has been a small but statistically significant increase in energy drink consumption among 18- to 35-year-olds.

Fulgoni noted several limitations to the NHANES survey data, including the self-report nature of the data, the lag between trends in the marketplace and data available to NHANES, and the small number of energy drink consumers.

Both Mitchell and Fulgoni emphasized the age dependency of caffeine exposure.

Methods

Mitchell described the study methodology and analysis. Data were collected from the Kantar Worldpanel Beverage Consumption Panel survey. Kantar Worldpanel is a global consumer panel company focused on the continuous measurement and analysis of consumer behaviors. This company has been conducting a continuous annual survey for more than 30 years, targeting U.S. consumers of all ages.

About 42,000 respondents were recruited from a panel of about 1 million people, with U.S. Census Bureau data used to ensure that the selection of participants was representative of the U.S. population. Sample selection criteria included age, gender, race, income, geographic region, household size, and presence of children in the household. Invitations were sent to English-speaking participants via e-mail and were staggered in batches sent weekly to ensure a balanced sample across all months of the year. Data were collected from the beginning of October 2010 through the end of September 2011. All panel participants were 1 year of age or older, with respondents consuming less than 21 beverages in 7 days excluded from the dataset.

Mitchell reported that participants were asked to begin completing their online surveys on a specific day for a total of 7 days. The online surveys required dragging and dropping beverage categories (soda/pop, hot coffee, iced coffee, milk, bottled water, and so forth) into different drinking occasion slots and then entering product details, including the type of beverage, amount consumed, where it was consumed, brand name, and other descriptive information. Beverages consumed both inside and outside the home were included. In addition, participants were asked to complete a "my info" questionnaire, which contained demographic, lifestyle, attitude, health, and nutrition questions. Height and weight data were also collected, with weight data for children collected for only 9 months of the 12-month data collection period (i.e., January through September 2011).

From this detailed beverage diary, Mitchell and colleagues were able to obtain a consolidated beverage list for each of the beverage categories (i.e., total beverages [i.e., all caffeinated beverages reported in the survey], carbonated soft drinks, energy drinks, energy shots, chocolate drinks, total coffee, total tea) and then, using the lists, develop a database. Developing the database required identifying which beverage categories contained beverages with caffeine. Information was obtained from manufacturers where possible, although the researchers also used a number of other resources as well. Mitchell emphasized that no single resource was comprehensive enough to capture information for all of the beverage and beverage types reported in the survey. Even the large national and research databases do not contain brand-specific data for the variety of beverages reported in the survey. The researchers assigned default values for beverages with no data available, insufficient detail, or no specified brand name. For example, the default value for a regular, brewed, nonspecialty brand of caffeinated coffee was 11.9 mg per fluid ounce. According to Mitchell, the range of default values reflects the variability in caffeine among different coffee types, with values ranging from 4.1 to 20.0 mg/fluid ounce for ready-to-drink bottle or canned coffee to 46.7 to 62.8 mg/fluid ounce for specialty espresso.

Once the database was developed, the researchers consolidated caffeine beverages into a more manageable set of categories for detailed analysis. The researchers were consistent with previous ILSI work with respect to the types of beverages included in each beverage category with one notable exception: energy drinks and energy shots were included as separate beverage categories. Neither was considered in the 1999 ILSI survey; energy drinks were not introduced into the market until 1997.

Although Mitchell and colleagues analyzed total caffeine intakes for all age groups across all categories, because coffee, carbonated soft drinks, tea, and energy drinks contributed approximately 98 percent or more of the caffeine consumed, Mitchell presented data only for those four categories.

The analysis covered only caffeinated beverage consumers, that is, consumers who drank 1 or more caffeinated beverages in 7 days, and only consumers 2 years of age and older. The researchers relied on parental reports for children, with two exceptions (i.e., data excluded from the analysis) to control for implausible survey entries: children with body weight data below the 3rd percentile or above the 97th percentile based on weight for age, using the Centers for Disease Control and Prevention (CDC) growth chart data as a reference, and children with total fluid intakes greater than two standard deviations above the mean fluid intake within a specific age year.

The small sample sizes for some subgroups in some beverage categories created another challenge. This was of particular concern for energy drinks for several age groups and for coffee for children between 2 and 5 years of age. In those cases, sample size was considered too small to provide reliable population estimates.

Results

Of the more than 42,000 survey respondents, 37,602 (85 percent) were caffeine consumers, that is, individuals who consumed at least one caffeinated beverage over a 7-day period of time (see Table 2-1). By age group, the proportion of the population consuming caffeine ranged from 43.0 percent in children 2 to 5 years of age to almost 100 percent of adults over the age of 65. This trend is consistent with previous reports in the literature, according to Mitchell.

Mean daily intake, expressed as both milligrams per day and milligrams per kilograms of body weight, steadily increased with age up to 65 years, when it fell slightly (see Table 2-1). The 50- to 64-year-old age group showed the highest intake. For the most part, the 90th percentile data follow the same trend. Again, the pattern is similar to what was reported almost a decade ago, although the intakes are higher. Mitchell noted that although there were some differences in mean daily intakes between men and women, the differences disappeared after adjusting for body weight.

When examined by beverage category, coffee, carbonated soft drinks, tea, and energy drinks together accounted for nearly all caffeine intake (see Table 2-2). As far as which type of beverage contributed the most, it was clearly coffee for all ages combined and for adults. For children, intakes were distributed fairly equally across coffee, carbonated soft drinks, and tea. Energy drinks contributed very little to beverage caffeine intakes.

TABLE 2-1 Number of Users and Mean and 90th Percentile Daily Intakes of Total Caffeinated Beverages, by Age

			Caffeine Intake			
Age Group (years)	No. of Users (sample size)	% Users (based on total U.S. population)	mg/day mean	mg/day 90th percentile	mg/kg/day mean	mg/kg/day 90th percentile
All ages	37,602	85.0	165±1	379.5	2.2±0.0	5.0
2–5	732	43.0	24±2	57.8	1.5±0.2	3.7
6–12	1,768	63.0	37±1	94	1.1±0.0	2.7
13–17	1,772	83.2	83±2	182.9	1.3±0.0	2.9
18–24	1,178	85.8	122±4	285.9	1.7±0.1	3.9
25–34	4,155	87.2	137±2	299.8	1.9±0.0	4.2
35–49	9,128	92.1	199±2	428.1	2.5±0.0	5.4
50–64	12,691	93.3	226±2	467.4	2.9±0.03	5.9
65 and older	6,178	99.6	207±2	419.9	2.6±0.03	5.4

SOURCE: Diane Mitchell. Presented to the Planning Committee for a Workshop on Potential Health Hazards Associated with Consumption of Caffeine in Food and Dietary Supplements on August 4, 2013.

Mitchell mentioned again that chocolate-containing beverages were not included in the data she presented because their contribution to total caffeine intake was so small, even though about 14 percent of the population surveyed reported consuming them. In the case of energy shots, the proportion of consumers in the sample was too low to estimate even when combining all ages. Together, chocolate-containing beverages and energy shots contributed less than 1 to 4 percent to total caffeine intake depending on age group. The amount of caffeine intake from those two categories is included in the estimates of the total caffeinated beverage category, however.

In order to understand more clearly what drives caffeine intake, Mitchell and colleagues examined caffeine intake within each beverage category for users only (i.e., users of that beverage category) (see Table 2-3). Among all ages, 55 percent of all caffeinated beverage consumers consumed coffee, 63 percent carbonated soft drinks, 53 percent tea, and 4 percent energy drinks. As an example of how to read Table 2-3, within the 50–64-year age group, 71 percent of caffeine users consumed coffee, with an estimated average daily intake among coffee users of 223 mg and a 90th percentile of 452 mg. Table 2-3 also shows where sample size was

TABLE 2-2 Mean Caffeine Intake by Age and Beverage Category

	Caffeine Intake (mg/day)				
Age Group (Years)	Total Caffeinated Beverages	Total Coffee	Total Carbonated Drinks	Total Tea	Total Energy Drinks
All ages	165±0.9	105±0.8	28±0.2	28±0.3	2.6±0.1
2–5	24±1.8	6±1.4	7±0.5	9.7±0.8	0.3±0.1
6–12	37±1.2	8±0.8	15±0.5	12±0.6	1.9±0.3
13–17	83±2.2	24±1.6	28±0.8	24±1.1	6.1±0.8
18–24	122±4.2	60±3.6	31±1.2	23±1.3	6.2±0.8
25–34	137±2.2	80±2	32±0.7	21±0.7	3.6±0.3
35–49	199±2.1	126±2.0	38±0.6	32±0.7	2.5±0.2
50–64	226±1.8	159±1.7	28±0.4	37±0.7	0.9±0.2
65 and older	207±2.3	159±2.2	16±0.4	32±0.7	0.9±0.2

NOTE: Total caffeinated beverages include carbonated soft drinks, energy drinks, total coffee, total tea, and a small percentage (1–4 percent depending on age group) from other sources (cocoa and chocolate-containing beverages, energy shots).
SOURCE: Diane Mitchell. Presented to the Planning Committee for a Workshop on Potential Health Hazards Associated with Consumption of Caffeine in Food and Dietary Supplements on August 4, 2013.

too low to obtain reliable estimates, which includes coffee among the youngest children and energy drinks among several age groups.

Summary of Caffeine Intake in the United States

In summary, caffeine intake in the United States comes primarily from four beverage types: coffee, tea, carbonated soft drinks, and energy drinks. In this recent ILSI survey, of those who reported consuming caffeinated beverages, more than half consumed each of three types of beverages (i.e., carbonated soft drinks [63 percent], coffee [55 percent], and tea [53 percent]), reflecting a significant number of caffeine consumers consuming more than one type of beverage. Although consumption of chocolate-containing beverages was high, the caffeine content of such beverages was low and contributed little to total caffeine intake.

TABLE 2-3 Caffeine Intakes for Users Within Each Beverage Category (mg/day)

	Coffee Drinkers (n=23,103)			Carbonated Soft Drink Drinkers (n=22,415)			Tea Drinkers (n=20,578)			Energy Drink Users (n=1,202)		
Age Group	% of users within age group	Mean daily intake	90th % intake	% of users within age group	Mean daily intake	90th % intake	% of users within age group	Mean daily intake	90th % intake	% of users within age group	Mean daily intake	90th % intake
All ages	55	191	394	63	45	102	53	53	126	4	60	144
2–5	7	—	—	51	13	34	45	22	56	1	—	—
6–12	10	76	179	70	21	51	39	29	69	4	—	—
13–17	27	92	224	77	37	80	53	45	104	10	59	133
18–24	46	130	288	70	45	99	54	43	110	9	—	—
25–34	53	153	316	68	46	108	52	41	98	6	60	160
35–49	61	209	418	66	57	127	52	61	145	4	63	149
50–64	71	223	452	57	49	109	57	65	153	2	58	126
65 and older	82	194	394	45	35	75	56	56	125	1	—	—

NOTE: Missing cells indicate where sample sizes were too low to obtain reliable estimates.
SOURCE: Diane Mitchell. Presented to the Planning Committee for a Workshop on Potential Health Hazards Associated with Consumption of Caffeine in Food and Dietary Supplements on August 4, 2013.

Mean daily caffeine intake was 165 mg. Intakes were higher than previously reported in the 1999 ILSI-sponsored beverage survey, when mean daily intake was 120 mg. The difference represents about half a cup of coffee or a can of carbonated soft drink. Mitchell cited several possible explanations for the increase. First, there were slightly more caffeine-consuming occasions reported in the more recent survey: 1.8 compared to 1.5. Second, there was a slight increase in the amount of coffee consumed (by fluid ounce) and a decrease in the amount of carbonated soft drinks consumed, and carbonated soft drinks have less caffeine. Third, the database values used for the more recent survey reflect higher caffeine values for specialty brand coffees, which may also have contributed.

A notable finding of the survey was the low consumption of energy drinks. Energy drinks were relatively new to the marketplace in 1999, and thus their intake was not estimated in the previous survey. So even though some energy drinks contain levels of caffeine similar to those of coffee, consumption of caffeine from energy drinks contributed little to total caffeine intake.

Caffeine intakes, in particular from coffee, for children between the ages of 2 and 12 years were higher than previously reported. But to keep that finding in perspective, Mitchell noted that only 9 percent of children between the ages of 2 and 12 years were reported to have consumed coffee.

Mean daily caffeine intake at the 90th percentile for all caffeinated beverages and among all ages was 380 mg or 5 mg per kg of body weight, most of which came from coffee. Daily caffeine intake at the 90th percentile for adults 35 years of age and older was slightly higher (420–467 mg/day) than the recommended maximum of 400 mg/day. Mitchell noted that the 400 mg/day threshold is not an official recommendation for caffeine in the United States. It is a Health Canada recommended level that is often used as a reference value. In addition, the FDA released two letters in 2012 stating that 400 mg per day was not associated with any adverse health effects and that the 400 mg per day value reflects recommendations set forth by Health Canada. For women of childbearing age (the 18- to 24-year-old and the 25- to 34-year-old age groups), both mean and 90th percentile caffeine intakes were below the <300 mg/day recommended levels for pregnancy. For children younger than 12 years of age and older children aged 13 to 17 years, 90th percentile intakes were slightly higher than the recommended 2.5 mg/kg/day.

In conclusion, as far as Mitchell was aware, the survey she described was the first population-based study in more than a decade to estimate caffeine intakes from beverages. The increase in accuracy afforded by the caffeine database developed for this study was a major strength, in Mitchell's opinion, although it may have contributed to the slightly higher caffeine intakes than previously reported. Overall, caffeine intakes remain largely driven by coffee consumption and, to a lesser extent, tea and carbonated soft drinks. Energy drink intakes contribute very little. In Mitchell's opinion, the data do little to support the notion that the introduction of additional caffeinated beverages into the marketplace has resulted in proportionately higher caffeine intakes by any of the various subpopulations of consumers.

VARIOUS ASPECTS OF CAFFEINE INTAKE IN AMERICA: ANALYSIS OF NHANES

Presented by Victor Fulgoni III, Ph.D.,
Nutrition Impact, LLC

Victor Fulgoni III described four ways that data from the National Health and Nutrition Examination Survey (NHANES) have been used to assess caffeine intake among Americans: (1) current usual intake of caffeine; (2) current usual intake of caffeine per consumption event; (3) trends in caffeine intake over the past decade; and (4) food sources of caffeine intake over the past decade. Data from multiple sets of surveys were used: 2001–2010 (N = 42,154) for the trend analyses and 2007–2010 (N = 17,387) for the intake analyses, with individuals under the age of 2 years and pregnant and/or lactating females excluded. Data include caffeine intake from all foods and beverages, but not dietary supplements.

To determine usual intake and usual intake per consumption event, Fulgoni and colleagues used the National Cancer Institute method (Tooze et al., 2010), which allows assessment of multiple days of intake and removal of intraperson variation. According to Fulgoni, the method provides a reasonable estimate of habitual chronic intake, which is what usual intake is intended to reflect. For trend data, Fulgoni and colleagues used 1-day intakes regressed over time, with $p < 0.01$ deemed significant.

Fulgoni reiterated what Mitchell had emphasized regarding evidence showing that more than 90 percent of the caffeine intake among Americans is from beverages, mostly coffee, tea, soda, and energy drinks. For coffee, caffeine levels included in the NHANES database range from 0.4 to 509 mg per reference amounts customarily consumed (RACCs). The

RACC for coffee is usually around 8 ounces. So, the range of caffeine levels is quite high, with the most frequently consumed coffee, that is, a typical brewed coffee, having 95 mg per RACC. For tea, the range is 0 to 48 mg/RACC, which covers all hot and cold tea beverages including zero-caffeine herbal tea. The most commonly consumed tea, a standard cup of leaf tea, has 48 mg/RACC. For soda, the range is 0 to 65 mg/RACC, with the most commonly consumed soda being a cola-type soda containing about 20 mg/RACC. Finally, for energy drinks included in the NHANES database, the range is 45 to 86 mg/RACC, with the most frequently consumed energy drink containing 72 mg/RACC.

Usual Intake

For caffeine consumption per day, among the total sample population (N = 17,387), mean intakes ranged from about 25 mg among 2- to 11-year-old children to more than 200 mg in older adults (see Figure 2-1). Among consumers only (N = 13,923), daily consumption ranged from less than 50 mg in 2- to 11-year-old children to more than 250 mg in the 50- to 59-year-old age group (see Figure 2-1).

Even at the 90th percentiles of intake, daily intake was only about 50 mg among young children (2 to 11 years) and barely more than 100 mg in adolescents (12 to 17 years) (see Figure 2-2). The highest-consuming age group, those 50 to 59 years of age, had a percentile intake of about 450 mg/day. Among consumers only, with the approximately 4,000 non-caffeine consumers removed from the dataset, the only age group that showed a noticeable difference from the total population 90th percentile intake was the 50- to 59-year-old age group, which jumps up to about 515 mg/day (see Figure 2-2). In sum, Fulgoni noted, for both mean usual intake and at the 90th percentile, caffeine intake is highly age-dependent. Both mean intake and the 90th percentile of intake were lowest in children 2 to 11 years and adolescents 12 to 17 years and highest in adults 50 to 59 years.

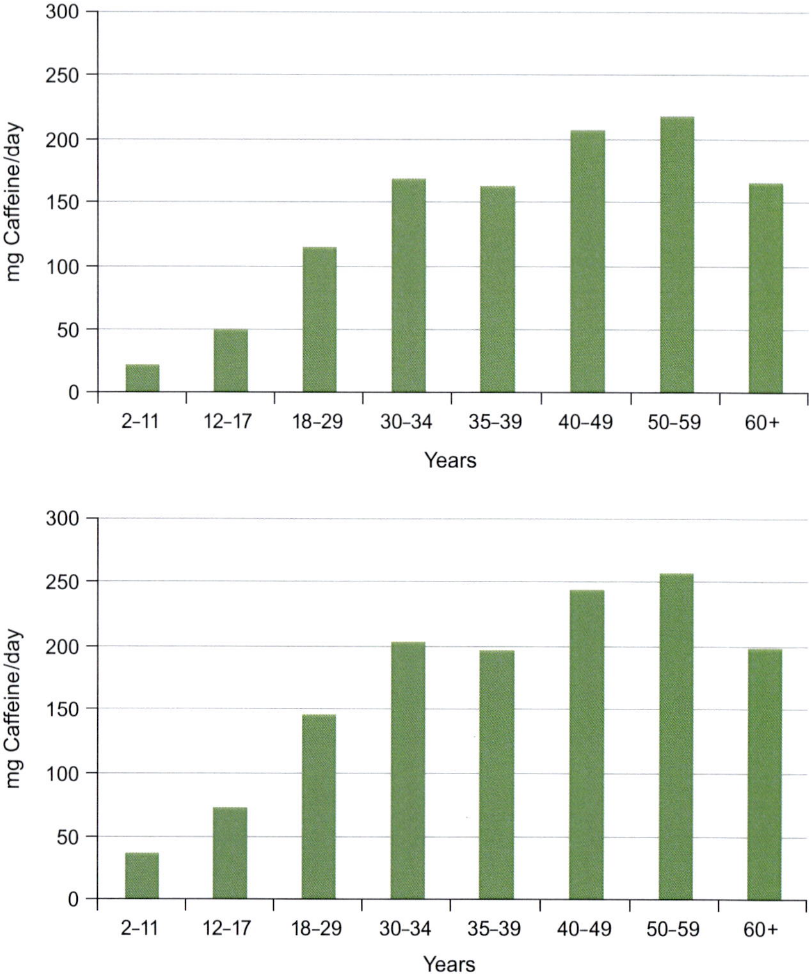

FIGURE 2-1 Mean usual intake of caffeine for total sample population (top) and caffeine consumers only (bottom).
SOURCE: NHANES.

Usual Intake by Consumption Event

A consumption event was defined as every time an individual consumed a food or beverage with caffeine, whether it was chocolate milk, coffee ice cream, coffee, an energy drink, cola, or something else. Again, both mean and the 90th percentile of usual intake per consumption event

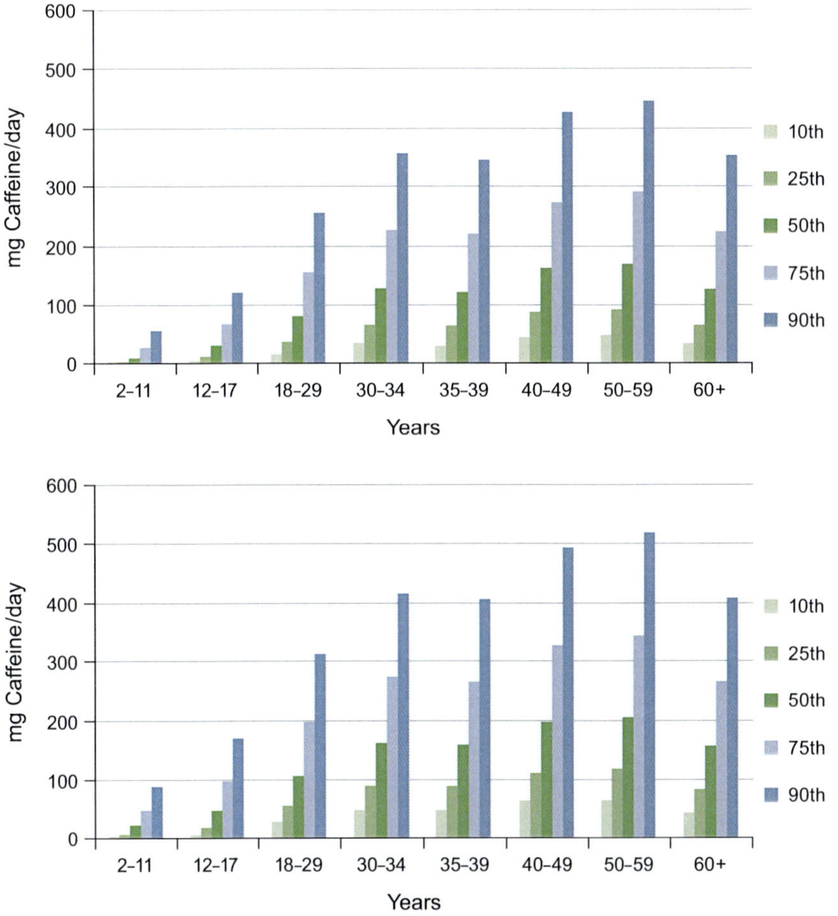

FIGURE 2-2 The 90th percentiles of usual caffeine intake for total sample population (top) and caffeine consumers only (bottom).
SOURCE: NHANES.

are highly age-dependent. The total population mean per consumption event was 65 mg. But among children 2 to 11 years, mean usual intake per consumption event was about 15 mg per event; among adolescents, it was about 35 mg; and among adults, it was 70 to 80 mg, depending on the age group (see Figure 2-3). At the 90th percentile, again, as with usual intake, among children the usual caffeine intake per consumption event was low: only about 25 mg, increasing to about 60 mg among adolescents and about 140 mg among adults (see Figure 2-3).

Trends in Caffeine Intake

Trends in caffeine intake data were assessed using single 24-hour recall information collected over time, using data from 2001 to 2010. Most age groups showed flat regression lines over time, meaning that

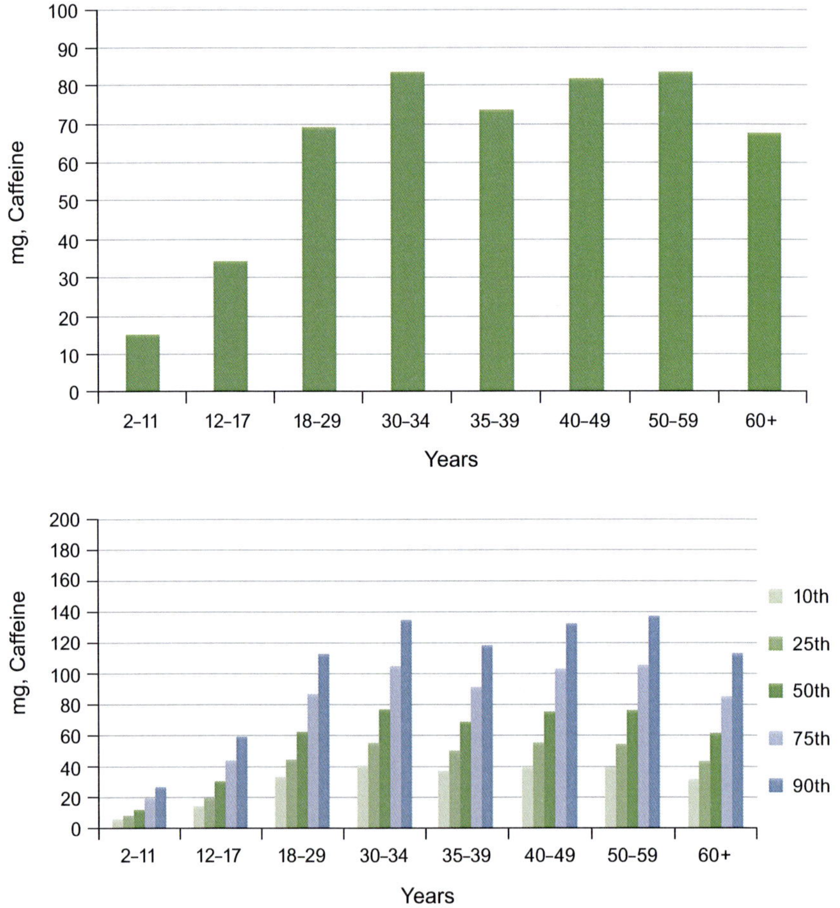

FIGURE 2-3 Mean and percentiles of usual caffeine intake (mg) per consumption event.
SOURCE: NHANES.

caffeine intake has remained relatively stable over the past decade. The only statistically significant regression coefficients were for the 2- to 11-year-old age group ($p < 0.01$) and the 35- to 39-year-old age group ($p < 0.01$). Both of those age group's regression coefficients were actually negative, suggesting slightly lower intake over time. For the 2- to 11-year-old age group, caffeine intake decreased about 2.5 mg on average per data release (i.e., data are released every 2 years); for the 35- to 39-year-old age group, it decreased about 19 mg on average per data release. In sum, intakes did not change much between 2001 and 2010. If anything, there were slight decreases in two age groups.

Trends in Caffeine Intake by Food Sources

Trends in caffeine intake by food sources were analyzed using the total sample population (thus not just consumers). For the 2- to 11-year-old age group, sodas, the major source of caffeine in that age group, showed a statistically significant downward trend in consumption from 2001 to 2010 ($p < 0.01$). The other beverage categories (coffee, tea, and energy drinks) showed no change over time. Fulgoni emphasized that one of the limitations of this analysis was the very low sample size for energy drinks.

In the 12- to 17-year-old age group, again soda was the major source of caffeine, and, again, it showed a statistically significant decline over time ($p < 0.01$). Caffeine intake from soda also decreased over time among the 18- to 35-year-old age group ($p < 0.01$). This is the only age group for which a statistically significant increase in energy drinks was observed ($p < 0.01$). Fulgoni noted that it was a small increase, but it was statistically significant. In the 51-years-and-older age group, despite being the highest caffeine consumers, researchers saw no change in intake by food source over time. Coffee remains by far the number-one source of caffeine in adults.

In sum, sodas are the largest source of caffeine in children 2 to 11 years and in adolescents (12 to 17 years). In both groups, caffeine intake from soda has actually decreased over the past decade. Coffee is the largest source of caffeine in adults. Energy drinks contribute little to the caffeine intake for any age group, although a small increase in intake (1 mg per 2-year data release) was detected for one age group.

Conclusion from the NHANES Analysis

With trends in caffeine intake remaining stable, or decreasing in some age groups, but with new sources of caffeine entering the marketplace, Fulgoni suggested that new sources of caffeine may be replacing older sources. Studies specifically designed to assess trade-off of caffeine sources would need to be conducted to confirm this suggestion.

Fulgoni concluded by remarking that, as is true of any study, there are strengths and limitations to these NHANES analyses. Their strengths are that they are based on a large nationally representative sample of children and adults and that usual intakes were analyzed using sophisticated statistical techniques. None of the data were adjusted for body size, although those data are available if necessary. Their limitations are that intake data were self-report; intake data were limited by what was available through NHANES (i.e., 2001–2010, with 2009–2010 the last publicly released data available); and some age groups had a small number of consumers of energy drinks.

PANELIST DISCUSSION WITH THE AUDIENCE

Following Fulgoni's presentation, workshop participants were invited to ask questions of the two panelists. This section summarizes the discussion that occurred. Most questions revolved around data and clarification of how those data have been analyzed and whether the same data can be analyzed in other ways to address additional questions, such as questions about vulnerable populations.

The 90th Percentile

The panelists were asked whether the data they presented allow for an examination of exposure among even heavier caffeine consumers—for example, consumers at the 95th or even 99th percentile. If not, are there other data available that can be used to examine exposure among the heaviest caffeine consumers in the population? Fulgoni replied that some intake estimates can be calculated at both the 95th and 99th percentiles, depending on gender and age.

Overweight and Obesity

There was some discussion about whether recent increases in overweight and obesity in the United States have implications with respect to the way caffeine is distributed in the body (e.g., in fat cells) and what the most appropriate metric is for evaluating or recommending dosage. Mitchell replied that estimates of caffeine exposure in terms of milligram per kilogram of body weight is probably not the best metric for heavier people if caffeine is not distributed in body fat the same way that it is distributed in lean mass. Fulgoni suggested that one possible solution might be to do what is done with protein recommendations, that is, use measure of height to determine ideal body weight (i.e., based on a 24.9 body mass index, or BMI) and then set a recommended exposure level on that basis.

Use of Averages to Estimate Caffeine Intake

Some participants expressed concern that "key facts" have been buried under the weight of averages, especially with respect to potentially vulnerable populations. For example, how many exposures of 150 mg, 200 mg, or 400 mg or more per event are occurring among adolescents yearly? And how has the number of those exposures changed over the years as the use of caffeine-containing energy drinks has increased? Mitchell and Fulgoni agreed that such an analysis could be done, for example, by analyzing consumption events per single day. Still, there might not be enough people consuming energy drinks to examine energy drink exposures in particular, depending on the age group. Fulgoni further remarked that the analyses he described were conducted before this workshop was conceived, and thus they did not separately examine pregnant and lactating women. But that group could be analyzed separately, he said.

The NHANES Database

One audience member asked Fulgoni whether the analyses he presented accounted for the fact that caffeine concentrations in products change over time. Fulgoni explained that all data releases are updated as necessary and that, in fact, one could use the NHANES database to analyze change in composition over time.

Another audience member asked about the accuracy of self-report data, especially with parents self-reporting consumption among their children. Fulgoni repeated that self-report is a limitation of the NHANES data. With respect to parental self-reporting of their children's consumption, parents report food and beverage consumption for children up to the age of 6 years. Between 6 years and 12 years, analysts use a combination of child and parental data. He was not aware of any study validating the NHANES self-report data for those younger ages.

Workshop planning committee chair Lynn Goldman commented on the number of new caffeinated products, such as candies and marshmallows, that are entering the marketplace and asked whether those types of products will be identifiable in the NHANES database in the future. Fulgoni replied that, although those specific products are not yet in the database, the product forms are. So, for example, marshmallows are in the database, making it possible to identify the age groups most likely to consume marshmallows and modeling intake on that basis.

Finally, Fulgoni highlighted the public availability of the NHANES database and remarked that any of his analyses could be repeated by others.

Dietary Supplement Exposure Among Fitness Enthusiasts

There was some discussion about caffeine use among individuals consuming sports nutrition supplements and whether that consumption might be skewing results for the intake of caffeine. Regan Bailey observed that when she dug into the NHANES database, she found only 17 reports of a caffeine-containing dietary supplement between 2007 and 2010. Fulgoni agreed that there is very little consumption of caffeine-containing dietary supplements. When asked whether the data he presented included Monster Energy consumption, given that Monster Energy was classified as a dietary supplement until recently, he replied "yes." If the interest is in sports and fitness, Fulgoni pointed out, it would be possible to analyze caffeine intake based on the activity metrics that are included in some of the NHANES datasets.

Energy Drink Marketing Data

Speaker John Higgins pointed out that marketing data indicate that 2.5 gallons of energy beverage per person, including babies and children, were consumed in the United States in 2009. He also observed that energy beverages are marketed very heavily to the teenage through 35-year-old age range. He asked, who is drinking all the energy beverages? Babies are clearly not drinking them, so who is? And is it possible that the data Mitchell and others are collecting are not capturing all energy beverage consumption events? He said he expected greater energy consumption events, given how marketing data indicate a high consumption of energy beverages. Mitchell reiterated that she and her colleagues found very low consumption. She suggested that the limitations of self-report data may have been a factor. Fulgoni observed that 2.5 gallons per year, or 320 ounces, amounts to less than an ounce a day, implying that it is not much. Higgins reiterated that the 2.5 gallons per year is across the total population and that some people consume more than others. Goldman pointed out the time lag between the NHANES data release and marketing data, noting that the NHANES data are "always a few years behind."

Addition or Substitution of Caffeine Sources?

The panelists were asked their thoughts on whether consumers are substituting new sources of caffeine for old sources or consuming multiple types of caffeine-containing foods and beverages. Mitchell observed that consumers are "obviously" consuming more than one type of caffeinated beverage. Although she and her colleagues did not separately examine multiple users—for example, to assess what and when they were consuming—the data are robust and could be analyzed to answer those types of questions. Likewise, with the NHANES database, according to Fulgoni, its robustness would allow for analyzing consumption of multiple types of beverages. He cautioned, however, that a robust estimate of energy drink consumption in children would probably require future oversampling.

REFERENCES

Knight, C. A., I. Knight, D. C. Mitchell, and J. E. Zepp. 2004. Beverage caffeine intakes in U.S. consumers and subpopulations of interest: Estimates from the Share of Intake Panel survey. *Food and Chemical Toxicology* 42:1923–1930.

Knight, C. A., I. Knight, and D. C. Mitchell. 2006. Beverage caffeine intakes in young children in Canada and the U.S. *Canadian Journal of Dietetic Practice and Research* 67:96–99.

Mitchell, D. C., C. A. Knight, J. Hockenberry, R. Teplansky, and T. J. Hartman. 2013. Beverage caffeine intakes in the U.S. *Food and Chemical Toxicology* S0278-6915(13)00717-5 63:136–142.

Tooze, J. A., V. Kipnis, D. W. Buckman, R. J. Carrolee, L. S. Freedman, P. M. Guenther, S. M. Krebs-Smith, A. F. Subar, and K. W. Dodd. 2010. A mixed-effects model approach for estimating the distribution of usual intake of nutrients: The NCI method. *Statistical Methods* 29(27):2857–2868.

3

Safety Signals and Surveillance

In addition to estimating exposure, another important first step to assessing the public health safety of the growing number of new caffeine-containing food and beverage products entering the marketplace is conducting surveillance and identifying incidents that warrant further investigation. The panelists of the Day 1, Session 2, panel, moderated by Steven E. Lipshultz, M.D., Department of Pediatrics, University of Miami, Florida, considered the types of surveillance in place and the safety signals being detected. This chapter summarizes their panel presentations and the discussion that followed. Box 3-1 describes the key points made by each speaker.

CAFFEINE AND ENERGY DRINK EXPOSURE CALL SURVEILLANCE

Presented by Alvin C. Bronstein, M.D., Rocky Mountain Poison Center

The United States, Puerto Rico, and the U.S. Virgin Islands, plus three Pacific jurisdictions, are served by 56 U.S. poison centers, with all the information from callers contemporaneously entered into a computer database and uploaded approximately every 19 minutes to the National Poison Data System (NPDS). Alvin C. Bronstein described the type of data collected during those calls and presented results from a descriptive analysis of caffeine exposure calls from January 2000 through July 2013 and energy drink exposure calls from June 2010 to July 2013.

BOX 3-1
Key Points Made by Individual Speakers

Alvin Bronstein described the National Poison Data System (NPDS), a near real- time national public health database, which collects call information from all 56 U.S. poison centers. Although centralized, national medical databases are not perfect, but they can nonetheless serve as a valuable resource for early safety signals. NPDS can provide critical insight into early recognition of trends in chemical, pharmaceutical, and commercial products including caffeine and energy drink exposures.

Bronstein presented the methods and results of a descriptive analysis of poison center calls showing an initial increase but recent stabilization in caffeinated energy product calls between 2010 and 2013. Bronstein opined that it is too early to predict future trends in energy product calls. Eighteen percent of the energy product calls resulted in no effect, with agitation, irritability, and tachycardia being the most frequently reported clinical effects.

In addition to serving as a resource for early safety signals, Bronstein emphasized, the U.S. National Poison Control Center database could be used for more systematic and prospective data collection and analysis related to caffeine exposure.

Ashley Roberts described how industry has used the GRAS process to determine the safety of caffeine as a food or beverage ingredient, including as an ingredient in energy drinks. In addition to NHANES data, industry has relied on data from a wealth of animal toxicity and human safety studies. He disparaged case reports publicized by the media that are not supported by the weight of scientific evidence.

Poison Center Calls and Data

Bronstein described the NPDS as a passive system, not an active system. Calls come from both consumers and health care professionals, with most centers using registered nurses or poison specialists to field the calls and others using PharmDs. All are backed by medical and clinical toxicologists or physicians. Poison centers field two types of calls: information calls, which are questions about substances, events, or medical conditions, and exposure calls. Data collected during the calls include information on 131 clinical effects, or "signs and symptoms," with all data collected since 2000 available online.

According to Bronstein, in addition to the contemporaneous recording of the calls by poison specialists, the poison centers also maintain a robust products database containing brand name and composition information for more than 390,000 products. The information typically comes directly from the companies that produce the products. Included are

4,401 caffeine products, 262 energy drinks, and 36 energy products (i.e., typically energy bars). The database can be searched by ingredient (e.g., taurine), as well as by product name.

Since 2000, poison centers have received about 2.5 million exposure calls per year (see Figure 3-1), with peak times consistently being June, July, and August (Bronstein et al., 2012). The change over time for various types of agents has been very consistent, according to Bronstein, with steady increases during the past 12 years in exposure calls related to analgesics, sedatives/hypnotics/antipsychotics, cardiovascular drugs, and antihistamines.

An Analysis of Caffeine-Related and Energy-Product Exposure Calls, 2000–2013

Bronstein described the methods and results from an analysis of single substance, closed, human exposure calls related to either caffeine (from January 1, 2000, through July 22, 2013) or energy products (from June 18, 2010, through July 22, 2013). For the purposes of the analysis, energy drinks and energy products were combined. July 22, 2013, was chosen as the end date because that was the day Bronstein and his colleagues started analyzing the data. The analysis of energy product calls began on June 18, 2010, because energy product generic codes were not added to the generic code vocabulary until mid-2010. (Products are categorized using a controlled hierarchical vocabulary, with seven energy product generic codes.) Bronstein and his colleagues calculated descriptive statistics; examined changes over time via either linear regression or spline fit; and correlated clinical effect frequencies. They used SAS JMP 9.0 for their analysis.

The researchers identified 48,177 caffeine calls between January 1, 2000, and July 22, 2013, and 6,724 energy product calls between June 18, 2010, and July 22, 2013. In these calls, the caller said that either the caller or his or her child or other person had ingested what was identified as either a product containing caffeine or an energy product.

As shown in Figure 3-2, caffeine exposure calls per day, by year, were not typical of the change over time that other products have shown over the past 12 years (i.e., as shown in Figure 3-1). Also shown in Figure 3-2, energy product exposure calls per day, by year, increased initially and then appeared to level off, although Bronstein stressed that it is too early to predict whether the leveling off will persist.

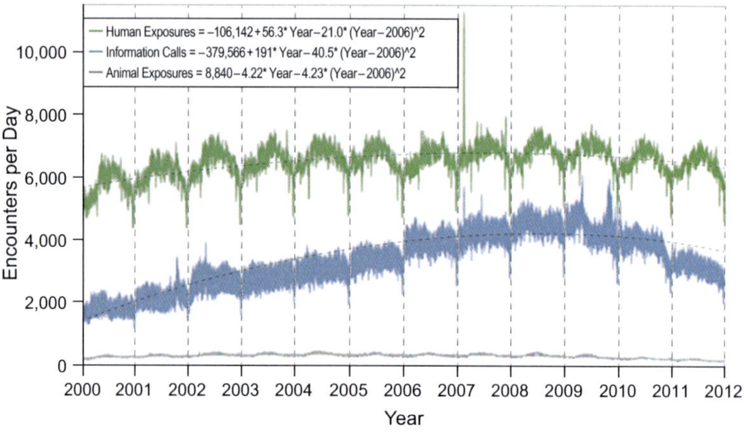

FIGURE 3-1 U.S. poison center calls per day, 2000–2012.
SOURCE: Bronstein et al., 2012.

Data on the total number of poison center calls received related to caffeine exposure were collected from January 1, 2000, through July 22, 2013, and calls related to energy product consumption from June 18, 2010, through July 22, 2013. Data were analyzed as change over time with linear regression, and correlation with clinical effect frequency. As shown in Table 3-1, of the 6,724 energy product calls analyzed, about 40 percent were for energy drinks containing caffeine only (i.e., without any other substance contributing to caffeine production, so no guarana, kola nut, tea, yerba mate, cocoa, and so forth). Initially, there were a small number of calls for energy drinks containing caffeine and ethanol (alcohol), an observation that led Bronstein to note that he and his colleagues have learned over the course of time that poison center calls can be used to show the effects of product withdrawals (i.e., energy drinks containing both alcohol and caffeine were withdrawn from the U.S. market after the FDA sent warning letters in 2010 to the manufacturers of those products).

With respect to reasons for energy product calls, most calls analyzed (55 percent) were unintentional. Unintentional calls are usually exposures in young children who do not demonstrate intent. The next two most common reasons for energy product calls were for intentional misuse (12 percent) and intentional abuse (8 percent).

With respect to age categories, the highest mean exposures per month were for children aged 2 years (26.50 mean exposures/month), children aged 6 to 12 years (17.50 mean exposures/month), and adults

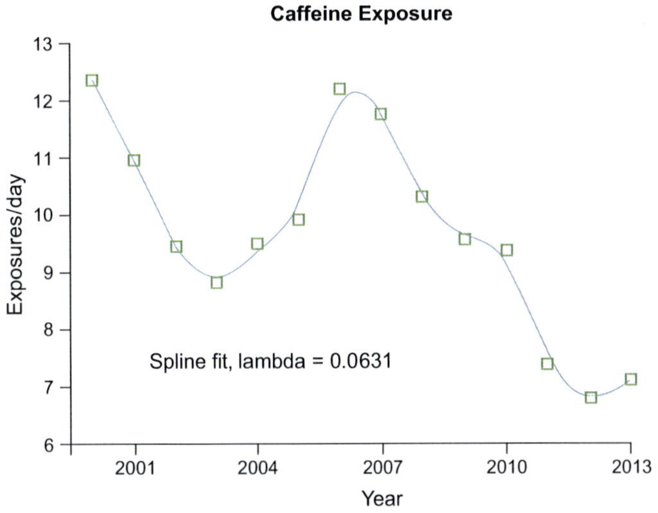

Year	Single
2000	4523
2001	3997
2002	3449
2003	3219
2004	3479
2005	3617
2006	4455
2007	4292
2008	3766
2009	3482
2010	3426
2011	2696
2012	2488
2013	1288
Total	48177

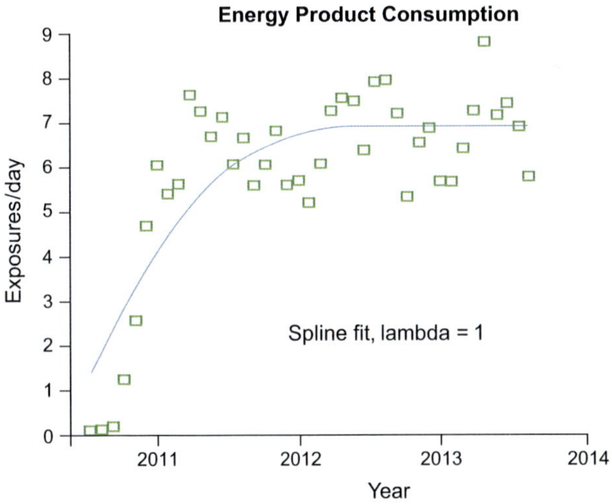

Year	Exposures
2010	496
2011	2309
2012	2471
2013	1448
Total	6724

FIGURE 3-2 Caffeine and energy product exposure calls per day over time.
SOURCE: Alvin Bronstein. Presented to the Planning Committee for a Workshop on Potential Health Hazards Associated with Consumption of Caffeine in Food and Dietary Supplements on August 4, 2013.

aged 20 to 59 years (42.00 mean exposures/month). Among the 2-year-old children, which Bronstein noted is a prime age for unintentional ingestion of substances, a linear regression revealed that the number of ingestions increased over time between June 18, 2010, and July 22, 2013, but with an r^2 value of only 0.41 ($p < 0.0001$).

Medical outcomes associated with energy product calls received are listed in Table 3-2. Bronstein highlighted that 18 percent of the 6,724 energy product calls between June 18, 2010, and July 22, 2013, showed no effect. About 10 percent had a moderate effect, which includes symptoms such as tachycardia. About 20 percent had minor effects—for example, hyperactivity or other effects that generally resolve. There was one death associated with consumption (2011). Among 2-year-old children, 34 percent of exposures had no effect, 12 percent had a minor effect, and only three children experienced what would be considered a moderate effect.

When Bronstein and colleagues compared the rank order of energy drink central nervous system clinical effects versus the rank order of central nervous system effects for all caffeine-related exposures, calls that did not involve energy products, they noticed similar patterns. For example, the most common central nervous system clinical effect, "agitated/irritable," for both types of calls ranked third among all clinical effects for energy drinks and fifth for other caffeine-related calls. The next

TABLE 3-1 Energy Product Calls by Generic Code, June 18, 2010, Through July 22, 2013

N	%	Energy Product Generic Code
2,664	39.6	Energy drinks: caffeine only (without guarana, kola nut, tea, yerba mate, cocoa, and so forth) (0200606)
1,870	27.8	Energy drinks: caffeine containing (from any source including guarana, kola nut, tea, yerba mate, cocoa, etc.) (0200605)
1,092	16.2	Energy drinks: unknown (0200608)
711	10.6	Energy products: other (0200609)
318	4.73	Energy drinks: ethanol and caffeine containing (from any source including guarana, kola nut, tea, yerba mate, cocoa, etc.) (0200610)
62	0.92	Energy drinks: no caffeine (from any source) (0200607)
7	0.10	Energy drinks: ethanol and caffeine only (without guarana, kola nut, tea, yerba mate, cocoa, etc.) (0200611)

SOURCE: Alvin Bronstein. Presented to the Planning Committee on Potential Health Hazards Associated with Consumption of Caffeine in Food and Dietary Supplements on August 4, 2013.

TABLE 3-2 Medical Outcomes for 6,724 Energy Product Calls Received Between June 18, 2010, and July 22, 2013

N	%	Medical Outcome
2,548	37.9	Not followed; minimal clinical effects possible (no more than minor effects possible)
1,301	19.3	Minor effect[a]
1,205	17.9	No effect
668	9.93	Moderate effect[b]
482	7.17	Unable to follow; judged as potentially toxic exposure
254	3.78	Not followed; judged as nontoxic exposure (clinical effects not expected)
216	3.21	Unrelated effect; exposure was probably not responsible for the effect(s)
29	0.43	Major effect[c]
20	0.30	Confirmed nonexposure
1	0.01	Death

NOTES: [a]minor effect = symptoms that generally resolve, for example, hyperactivity; [b]moderate effect = possible harm with symptoms such as tachycardia; [c]major effect = serious harm or death.
SOURCE: Alvin Bronstein. Presented to the Planning Committee for a Workshop on Potential Health Hazards Associated with Consumption of Caffeine in Food and Dietary Supplements on August 4, 2013.

most common central nervous system clinical effect for both types of calls, "dizziness/vertigo," ranked seventh among clinical effects for energy drink calls and eighth for caffeine calls. Next for both types of calls was "tremor," followed by "headache." In a similar comparison of the rank order of cardiovascular effects, again there appeared to be a good correlation in rank order between the two types of calls. The most common cardiovascular effect, tachycardia, ranked fourth for both energy drink and caffeine calls. The overall correlation of clinical effect frequencies (i.e., all clinical effects recorded) between energy product and caffeine exposure calls was 0.942 ($p < 0.0001$) (Bronstein et al., 2012). Bronstein remarked that he and his colleagues would like to investigate this trend more thoroughly in an effort to identify which components of energy products are responsible for the clinical effects so similar to those being seen with caffeine exposure calls.

Conclusions About Energy Drink Exposure Calls

In summary, energy product exposure calls to U.S. poison centers initially increased but appear to have stabilized, although without a full year (2013) of data, it is difficult to know whether the trend has in fact stabilized. Most energy product exposure calls are unintentional, followed by misuse and abuse. The most frequently reported clinical effects were agitation, irritability, and tachycardia. But 18 percent of energy product calls were recorded as having no effect. Bronstein and his colleagues believe that the energy product clinical effect pattern is very similar to that of caffeine ingestions, but more work in that area needs to be done. Similarly, although poison center data allow for analysis of calls by specific active agents, more work in that area needs to be done as well.

Limitations of poison center data include the fact that they represent self-reported exposures, whether from health care professionals or the public, so underreporting is likely. Also, exposures are confirmed with clinical laboratory data but only when clinically indicated. Generally, calls are not confirmed.

On the basis of his and his colleagues' findings, Bronstein made several recommendations for moving forward. Poison centers can assist with data gathering on energy product and caffeine exposure calls by (1) developing a prospective-focused system for data collection in collaboration with the FDA and the IOM; (2) focusing further analyses and surveillance on products with specific active ingredients (e.g., taurine-containing energy products), on vulnerable populations, and on clinical effect profiles of substances (e.g., via cluster analysis); and (3) providing real-time alerts of exposure calls of public health significance.

SAFETY ASSESSMENT OF CAFFEINE IN FOODS AND BEVERAGES

Presented by Ashley Roberts, Ph.D.,
Intertek Cantox

The industry approach to supporting the safety of food and beverage ingredients, such as caffeine, which includes energy drinks, relies on the GRAS determination process. Ashley Roberts provided an overview of the GRAS process as it pertains to caffeine and briefly considered some current international regulatory positions on the safety of energy drinks.

The GRAS Determination Process

The procedure of establishing the use of a substance as GRAS is FDA regulated. The GRAS status of a food ingredient is based on the consensus of experts qualified by scientific training and experience to evaluate its safety. GRAS status determination requires the same quality and quantity of scientific evidence needed to obtain food additive approval from the FDA, with the major difference being that the safety data used to determine GRAS status must be generally available to the scientific community. Equally important, Roberts said, the mere showing of safety is not sufficient. Rather, the use of the ingredient must be generally recognized as safe, which is normally achieved through publication of research in peer-reviewed journals.

Estimating Human Exposure

A key component in the safety evaluation process is estimating human exposure. According to Roberts, estimates of caffeine consumption can be calculated using the NHANES database.[1] On the basis of the data from the 2007–2008 and 2009–2010 NHANES surveys, 348 mg is the estimated daily intake at the 90th percentile for caffeine from background diet (i.e., caffeine in coffee) plus caffeine from energy drinks (i.e., at an incorporation level of up to 120 mg/8 ounces) and dietary supplements for the entire population. The highest estimated daily intake for caffeine from background diet plus energy drinks and dietary supplements at the 90th percentile is for male adults: 444 mg caffeine/day. Roberts observed that, compared to estimates for background exposures, adding energy drinks and dietary supplements to the diet results in a minimal increase in caffeine intake. Roberts noted that the 90th percentile is an FDA benchmark for high consumers and that, other than for male adults, estimates of caffeine intake at the 90th percentile among all other

---

[1]See Chapter 2 for a discussion of how the NHANES database has been used to estimate caffeine exposure among different age groups and changes in caffeine exposure over time.

groups are below the 400 mg safety threshold level indicated by the FDA to be a safe level.

Roberts identified several limitations of the NHANES database. First, the intake methodology generally overestimates exposure by assuming that all energy drink products in the marketplace have caffeine incorporated at the maximum use level. Exposures are further overestimated by assuming that consumption on a given day is always associated with consumption of caffeine from other sources, including dietary supplements, which may not be the case in real-life situations. Also, the NHANES food survey is a short-term survey over 2 days, which overestimates consumption over the longer term. Despite these limitations, exposure results from NHANES data are similar to those obtained from postmarketing surveillance data, including data from surveys conducted by the FDA and on behalf of the International Life Science Institute (RSEQ, 2011; FDA, 2012; ISQ, 2012; Mitchell et al., 2013). Moreover, two of those other surveys (RSEQ, 2011; ISQ, 2012), both conducted in Canada, collected data on up to 70,000 teenagers, showing that energy drink consumption 4 times or more weekly was found in about 2 percent of subjects, consistent with what the NHANES survey found.

Safety Data

The GRAS determining process for the safe use of caffeine as an added ingredient of food and beverages takes into account a range of data and information from metabolic, pharmacokinetic, animal, and human studies, including data on carcinogenicity, cardiovascular effects, seizures, and other specific effects and data on children and adolescents. Roberts highlighted studies that he thought most relevant.

With respect to the metabolism and pharmacokinetics of caffeine, Kempf et al. (2010) reported that high daily intakes of caffeine from coffee, up to 1 gm/day, do not result in bioaccumulation. Arnaud (2011) reported that caffeine kinetics appears to follow a first-order process, and Hodgson et al. (2013) demonstrated that the kinetics of naturally occurring caffeine in coffee is similar to those of anhydrous caffeine. Roberts remarked that the latter finding was especially interesting because anhydrous caffeine is what is added to products such as energy drinks.

Roberts noted that because the major metabolites produced in humans are almost identical to those found in rodents, this finding supports the use of rodents as animal models for assessing human safety. A complete range of toxicity studies has been conducted with animal models, with a no-observed-adverse-effect level (NOAEL) of approximately 100 mg per kg per day for carcinogenicity and reproductive effects (Brent et al., 2011). According to Roberts, that dose is considerably higher than what humans are exposed to on a daily basis and equates to somewhere in the region of 40 to 80 cups of coffee per day.

Human studies suggest that toxic doses of caffeine range from 3 g in young children to 10 g in adults (Iserson, 1990; Nawrot et al., 2003), which is equivalent to the consumption of between 28 and 93 8-ounce servings of energy drinks per day. With respect to specific effects, according to Roberts, caffeine has not been consistently linked with any adverse reproductive consequences. Nevertheless, both the European Commission's Scientific Committee on Food and Health Canada recommend that the consumption of caffeine during pregnancy be no more than 300 mg per day. To support these recommendations, energy drink companies have labeled their products as not being recommended for pregnant and nursing mothers.

With respect to carcinogenic potential, the International Agency for Research on Cancer has concluded that there is inadequate evidence to confirm that caffeine, as present in coffee, is carcinogenic, a viewpoint that has been confirmed in several large prospective trials (Nawrot et al., 2003; Nkondjock, 2009; Freedman et al., 2012). Roberts noted that, interestingly, the largest prospective study to date (Freedman et al., 2012), with roughly 620,000 subjects, included about 10,000 men and 5,000 women who consumed at least 6 cups of coffee per day, which Roberts opined could result in consumption levels far greater than 1 g caffeine per day.

Human studies on cardiovascular effects have shown that, while caffeine produces a slight but transient increase in blood pressure, other electrocardiogram parameters are not affected. Several reports, including recent meta-analyses of prospective studies, have concluded that the effects of caffeine on cardiovascular function are not clinically significant (IOM, 2001; Pelchovitz and Goldberger, 2011; Bohn et al., 2012; Freedman et al., 2012; Mostofsky et al., 2012). Similarly, for cardiac arrhythmias, results have shown that normal daily caffeine consumption, even when administered as a bolus dose in persons with arrhythmias, was well tolerated (Myers and Reeves, 1991; Pelchovitz and Goldberger, 2011; Menzes et al., 2013). Nevertheless, conflicting results have been reported among excessive consumers of coffee (i.e., more than nine cups per day) (Frost and Vestergaard, 2005; Gronroos and Alonso, 2010).

Although a number of case reports regarding seizures may be linked to energy drink consumption (e.g., Iyadurai and Chung, 2007; Trabulo et al., 2011), Roberts opined that these case reports have significant limitations that preclude establishing causality. A large and robust prospective study using data from the Nurses' Health Study cohort did not identify caffeine as a risk factor for developing seizure (Dworetsky et al., 2010).

Human studies have shown that acute caffeine administration negatively impacts calcium balance and glucose tolerance. Studies also show, however, that the effects on calcium balance can be mitigated through consumption of calcium in the diet (van Dam et al., 2004; Roberts and Rogerson, 2008; Bhupathiraju et al., 2013). Similarly, evidence from prospective studies suggests that caffeine from coffee protects against the risk of type 2 diabetes, thereby mitigating the short-term effects on glucose tolerance (Huxley et al., 2009; Wedick et al., 2011; Freedman et al., 2012; Bhupathiraju et al., 2013).

Available evidence from studies in children (12 years and younger) and adolescents suggests that caffeine results in similar pharmacokinetic and pharmacodynamic effects in younger individuals as those observed in adults (ANZFA, 2000; Meltzer et al., 2008). According to Roberts, the effects of caffeine are therefore considered to be more a function of body weight rather than age. Health Canada has suggested that caffeine consumption by children be limited to no more than 2.5 mg per kg body weight per day (Nawrot et al., 2003; Rotstein et al., 2013). Roberts remarked that caffeine has a long history of safe use in children for the treatment of apnea or prematurity and attention deficit disorder.

In the case of caffeine use in energy drinks, GRAS determinations have also taken into consideration potential interactions with alcohol. Although some researchers have hypothesized that caffeine may antagonize the effects of alcohol, resulting in greater alcohol consumption, the European Scientific Committee on Food and the UK Committee on Toxicity of Chemicals in Food Consumer Products and the Environment have reported that the totality of evidence is currently insufficient to conclude that co-consumption of energy drinks with alcohol is unsafe (SCF, 2003; COT, 2012).

In Roberts's opinion, the increasing concerns being expressed regarding the use of caffeine in energy drinks come from a number of case reports. All published case reports, however, including incidences of adverse events reported in the FDA's Adverse Event Reporting System[2] database, have been reviewed as part of the GRAS determination process. The expert panels reviewing this information agreed with the FDA's position that an adverse effect report itself reflects only information as reported and does not represent any conclusion regarding a causal relationship with the product or ingredient. Roberts pointed out that, in addition, the Drug Abuse Warning Network (DAWN) report called into question the causal link between energy drink consumption and emergency room visits because of a number of limitations in the data (SAMHSA, 2013).

In sum, according to Roberts, on the basis of an overall assessment of the safety information, experts have determined that there is no difference in the systematic handling of naturally occurring caffeine and caffeine added to foods and beverages, such as energy drinks. Nor is the premise that adolescents react differently than adults following caffeine consumption supported by the scientific evidence. Roberts noted that the caffeine content in energy drinks is similar to or below that of a number of marketed coffee products and the incremental use of caffeine in energy drinks combined with other sources of caffeine results in total human caffeine exposures below 400 mg/day in all age groups besides adult males. International regulatory positions, including those of the FDA and Health Canada, indicate that caffeine intake up to 400 mg daily is not associated with adverse effects.

In Roberts's opinion, the concern about caffeinated energy drinks is based on case reports that have been publicized in the media and are not supported by the weight of published scientific evidence on caffeine. The scientific experts who reviewed this evidence thought that the case reports were of limited relevance to a GRAS determination process and that the weight of scientific evidence, in combination with exposure data, supports the safety of caffeine in food and beverage products such as energy drinks.

PANELIST DISCUSSION WITH THE AUDIENCE

Following Roberts's presentation, the moderator invited the workshop audience to ask questions of either panelist. Most of the discussion

---

[2]The FDA's Adverse Event Reporting System is a computerized information database designed to provide support for postmarketing safety surveillance for all approved drug and therapeutic biologic products.

revolved around the interpretation of poison center data and the potential for future analyses of those data; the idea of a national registry to track health outcomes related to caffeine-containing energy drink exposure; the lack of data on interactions between caffeine and other ingredients in energy drinks (which is the subject of Chapter 6); and limitations of the available data.

Questions About Poison Center Data

There was some confusion about the reasons for poison center calls being categorized as intentional (misuse or abuse) versus unintentional. For example, how is intentional misuse different from unintentional use? Bronstein explained that an example of intentional misuse would be somebody consuming two or three doses of a product when the directions indicated that only one dose should be consumed. Intentional abuse would be the use of a drug or nondrug product for pharmacological effect or intoxication.

There were questions about reporting and whether the analysis that Bronstein presented included reports from both consumers and health care professionals. Bronstein said that the analysis did include both. Most health care professional reports are from emergency department physicians. He observed that, in general, calls from emergency departments are increasing for all substances. Although he and his colleagues did not examine emergency department data specifically, he said, it could be done.

Finally, there was some discussion about the 18 percent of no-effect cases that Bronstein described. An audience member described that specific conclusion as "misleading" because it implied that essentially 82 percent of cases had an effect. However, according to the audience member, on closer examination of children aged 12 years and younger, when cases that were not followed are included, in fact about 82 percent of cases in the pediatric population were asymptomatic and only 18 percent showed symptoms, the majority of which were minor. Bronstein explained that the 18 percent figure he reported was just one piece of information, that is, that 18 percent of all cases, including both pediatric and adult cases, were recorded as no effect. The audience member suggested that pulling and displaying data for children only, that is, for the pediatric population, would be helpful.

When asked how helpful it will be in the future to incorporate into the NPDS information on habitual versus nonhabitual use of caffeine, as well as information on actual caffeine levels, Bronstein replied that that type of information could certainly be collected. Currently, exposures are assigned chronicity, acute, acute-on-chronic, chronic, or unknown. Call history is taken in a manner similar to how physicians talk to their patients, with everyone doing it a little differently. In his opinion, the dataset could be standardized further to collect additional data.

Underreporting and the Need for a National Registry

Bronstein's mention (during his presentation) of underreporting prompted an audience member to observe that, when looking for information on myocardial infarctions, it became evident that not all emergency departments were capturing those data. Thus, a registry was developed and is now very well established within the United States such that anyone who experiences a myocardial infarction is well documented. Bronstein was asked whether a similar nationwide registry to track exposures and health outcomes might be beneficial in terms of "getting closer to the actual real data." Bronstein replied, "Absolutely." He remarked that the beginnings of such a registry already exist. Ninety-five percent of callers to poison centers provide phone numbers. If a nationwide registry could be structured, it would not be difficult to call those callers back and provide them with the option of being entered into a national registry. A national registry would be especially helpful for obtaining information on the effects of chronic exposures.

The Interaction Between Caffeine and Other Ingredients in Caffeine-Containing Energy Drinks

Roberts was asked to describe studies on interactions between caffeine and taurine, which the questioner noted seems to be a popular ingredient in energy drinks, or with any of the other chemical and herbal ingredients in energy drinks. Roberts replied that there are no data on the combination toxicology of the various ingredients in energy drinks. Having said that, all of the other ingredients have undergone the GRAS determination processes. With respect to taurine in particular, he noted that taurine occurs naturally in the diet and is a component of meat, poultry, seafood, and dairy products. It is also present in human breast milk and is added to some infant formulas. The level of taurine in energy drinks has been evaluated in the context of that background exposure scenario and is considered safe.

The Importance of Anecdotal Experience

An audience member disagreed with Roberts's remark during his presentation that case studies are irrelevant and argued that anecdotal experience helps to generate hypotheses.

Use of Animal Models to Study the Effects of Caffeine

Session 4 (Day 1) speaker Sergi Ferré commented on Roberts's claim that caffeine metabolites in rats versus humans are the same and that rats therefore serve as a good model for studying the safety of caffeine exposure in humans. He noted that paroxetine, a caffeine metabolite with very strong psychostimulant effects, is a much more active metabolite in humans than it is in rats.

Limitations of the Data

An audience member who described himself as a practicing board-certified emergency physician remarked that he has not been seeing serious side effects from caffeine from any source other than with intentional overdose from over-the-counter pills. He suggested that the approximately 6 billion energy drinks being sold every year in the United States, with an average of only about 2,000 calls per year to poison centers, almost none of which report serious side effects, is pretty strong evidence that energy drinks are in fact very safe products.

Bronstein replied, "Let the data speak for themselves." Whether the level of analysis he and his colleagues conducted for the purposes of this workshop, with the data they had, presents a "total picture" is unclear at this point. Furthermore, he noted that more studies are needed to determine what, if any, clinical effects are related to caffeine-containing energy drink exposures.

Audience members also offered some additional comments about the limitations of all datasets and how different datasets can lead to slightly different conclusions. For example, Session 3 (Day 2) panelist Steven

Lipshultz pointed out that the DAWN data suggest that the rate of adverse effects, as indicated by emergency room visits following energy drink exposure, is slightly higher than what the poison center data suggest. In response, another audience member commented that, even with the DAWN data, a numerator of approximately 10,000 (i.e., half of the approximately 20,000 emergency visits were for energy drink exposures alone, that is, not in combination with alcohol or another toxic ingestion) over an estimated 130 million emergency room visits per year suggests that the evidence for serious side effects is lacking. Lipshultz opined that, to the contrary, the DAWN data, as well as NHANES, ILSI, and poison center data, all point to the need for a more formal assessment. Each dataset has its limitations, but each also has it strengths. They all deserve further discussion.

REFERENCES

ANZFA (Australia New Zealand Food Authority). 2000. *Report from the Expert Working Group on the Safety Aspects of Dietary Caffeine*. Canberra, Australia/Wellington, New Zealand. http://foodsafety.govt.nz/elibrary/industry/ caffein-info-sheet.pdf (accessed November 26, 2013).

Arnaud, M. J. 2011. Pharmacokinetics and metabolism of natural methylxanthines in animal and man. *Handbook of Experimental Pharmacology* (200):33–91.

Bhupathiraju, S. N., A. Pan, V. S. Malik, J. E. Manson, W. C. Willett, R. M. van Dam, and F. B. Hu. 2013. Caffeinated and caffeine-free beverages and risk of type 2 diabetes. *American Journal of Clinical Nutrition* 97:155–166.

Bohn, S. K., N. C. Ward, J. M. Hodgson, and K. D. Croft. 2012. Effects of tea and coffee on cardiovascular disease risk. *Food and Function* 3(6):575–591.

Brent, R. L., M. S. Christian, and R. M. Diener. 2011. Evaluation of the reproductive and developmental risks of caffeine. *Birth Defects Research. Part B, Developmental and Reproductive Toxicology* 92:152–187.

Bronstein, A. C., D. A. Spyker, L. R. Cantilena, B. H. Rumack, and R. C. Dart. 2012. 2011 annual report of the American Association of Poison Control Centers' National Poison Data Systems (NPDS): 29th annual report. *Clinical Toxicology* 50:911–1164.

COT (Committee on Toxicity of Chemicals in Food, Consumer Products, and the Environment). 2012. *COT statement on the interaction of caffeine and alcohol and their combined effects on health and behavior*. http://cot.food.gov.uk/pdfs/cotstatementcaffalco201204.pdf (accessed December 25, 2013).

Dworetzky, B. A., E. B. Bromfield, M. K. Townsend, and J. H. Kang. 2010. A prospective study of smoking, caffeine, and alcohol as risk factors for seizures or epilepsy in young adult women: Data from the Nurses' Health Study II. *Epilepsia* 51:198–205.

FDA (U.S. Food and Drug Administration). 2012. *FDA comments on "Caffeine Intake by the U.S. Population," prepared by Laszlo P. Somogyi, 2010.* Silver Spring, MD: U.S. Food and Drug Administration, Center for Food Safety and Applied Nutrition, Oakridge National Laboratory. http://www.fda.gov/downloads/AboutFDA/Centers/Offices/OfficeofFoods/CFSAN/CFSANFOIAElectronicReadingRoom/UCM333191.pdf (accessed November 26, 2013).

Freedman, N. D., Y. Park, C. C. Abnet, A. R. Hollenbeck, and R. Sinha. 2012. Association of coffee drinking with total and cause-specific mortality. *New England Journal of Medicine* 366:1891–1904.

Frost, L., and P. Vestergaard. 2005. Caffeine and risk of atrial fibrillation or flutter: The Danish diet, cancer, and health study. *American Journal of Clinical Nutrition* 81(3):578–582.

Gronroos, N. N., and A. Alonso. 2010. Diet and risk of atrial fibrillation—epidemiological and clinical evidence. *Circulation Journal* 74:2029–2038.

Hodgson, A. B., R. K. Randell, and A. E. Jeukendrup. 2013. The metabolic and performance effects of caffeine compared to coffee during endurance exercise. *PloS ONE* 8(4):e59561.

Huxley, R., C. M. Lee, F. Barzi, L. Timmermeister, S. Czernichow, V. Perkovic, D. E. Grobbee, D. Batty, and M. Woodward. 2009. Coffee, decaffeinated coffee, and tea consumption in relation to incident type 2 diabetes mellitus: A systematic review with meta-analysis. *Archives of Internal Medicine* 169:2053–2063.

IOM (Institute of Medicine). 2001. *Caffeine for the sustainment of mental task performance: Formulations for military operations.* Washington, DC: National Academy Press.

Iserson, K. V. 1990. Caffeine and nicotine. In *Clinical management of poisoning and drug overdose*, 2nd ed., edited by L. M. Haddad and J. F. Winchester. Philadelphia, PA: W.B. Saunders Co. Pp. 869–876.

ISQ (Institute de la Statistique du Quebec). 2012. *Tableau A3.2: Frequence de consummation habituelle de certaines boissons sucrees, eleves du secondaire, Quebec, 2010–2011. Dans: L'Enquete quebecoise sur la santé des jeunes du secondaire 2010–2011: TOME 1: Le visage des jeunes d'aujourd'jui: leur santé physique et leurs habitudes ve vie.* Chemin Sainte-Foy, Quebec: Institut de la Statistique du Quebec. http://www.stat.gouv.qc.ca/publications/sante/eqsijs.htm (accessed November 26, 2013).

Iyadurai, S. J., and S. S. Chung. 2007. New-onset seizures in adults: Possible association with consumption of popular energy drinks. *Epilepsy and Behavior* 10:504–508.

Kempf, K., C. Herder, I. Erlund, H. Kolb, S. Martin, M. Carstensen, W. Koenig, J. Sundvall, S. Bidel, S. Kuha, and J. Tuomilehto. 2010. Effects of coffee consumption on subclinical inflammation and other risk factors for type 2 diabetes: A clinical trial. *American Journal of Clinical Nutrition* 91:950–957.

Meltzer, H. M., T. O. Fotland, J. Alexander, E. Elind, H. Hallstrom, H. R. Lam, K.-H. Liukkonen, M. A. Petersen, and E. J. Solbergsdottir. 2008. *Risk assessment of caffeine among children and adolescents in the Nordic countries*. Copenhagen, Denmark: Nordic Council of Ministers, TemaNord. http://www.nrden.org/en/publications/publikationer/2008-551/at_download/publicationfile (accessed November 26, 2013).

Menzes, A. R., C. L. Lavie, J. J. DiNicolantonio, J. O'Keefe, D. P. Morin, S. Khatib, and R. V. Milani. 2013. Atrial fibrillation in the 21st century: A current understanding of risk factors and primary prevention strategies. *Mayo Clinic Proceedings* 88(4):394–409.

Mitchell, D. C., C. A. Knight, J. Hockenberry, R. Teplansky, and T. J. Hartman. 2013. *Caffeine intakes from beverages in the U.S.* Abstract. http://www.fasebj.org/cgi/content/meeting_abstract/27/1_MeetingAbstracts/848.18?sid+eb47194e-54d1-40cb-b977-a6dfbd25280a (accessed November 26, 2013).

Mostofsky, E., M. S. Rice, E. B. Levitan, and M. A. Mittleman. 2012. Habitual coffee consumption and risk of heart failure: A dose-response meta-analysis. *Circulatory Heart Failure* 5(4):401–405.

Myers, M., and R. Reeves. 1991. The effect of caffeine on daytime ambulatory blood pressure. *American Journal of Hypertension* 4:427–431.

Nawrot, P., S. Jordan, J. Eastwood, J. Rotstein, A. Hugenholtz, and M. Feeley. 2003. Effects of caffeine on human health. *Food Additive and Contaminants* 20:1–30.

Nkondjock, A. 2009. Coffee consumption and the risk of cancer: An overview. *Cancer Letters* 277:121–125.

Pelchovitz, D. J., and J. J. Goldberger. 2011. Caffeine and cardiac arrhythmias: A review of the evidence. *American Journal of Medicine* 124(4):284–289.

Roberts, A., and R. Rogerson. 2008. Chinese approach on regulating food additives, novel foods, functional foods and dietary supplements. In *Nutraceutical and functional food regulations in the United States and around the world*, edited by D. Bagchi. New York: Elsevier. Pp. 291–303.

Rotstein, J., J. Barber, C. Stowbridge, H. Hayward, R. Huang, and S. Benrejeb Godefroy. 2013. Energy drinks: An assessment of the potential health risks in the Canadian context. *International Food Risk Analysis Journal* 3(4):1–29. http://cdn.intechopen.com/pdfs/45380/InTech-Energy_drinks_as_assessment_of_the_potential_health_risks_in_the_canadian_context.pdf (accessed November 26, 2013).

RSEQ (Reseau du sport etudiant du Quebec). 2011. *Enquete Quebecoise sur le marketing de la malbouffe: 10,000 jenunes se prononcent.* http://ll.rseq.ca/download/attachments/15958040/Rapport+d'enquete-FRA-1-page.pdf?version=1&modificationDate=1328122709903 (accessed November 26, 2013).

SAMHSA (Substance Abuse and Mental Health Services Administration). 2013. *The DAWN report.* http://www.samhsa.gov/data/Short_Reports.aspx (accessed November 26, 2013).

SCF (Scientific Committee on Food). 2003. *Opinion of the Scientific Committee on Food (SCF) on additional information on "energy" drinks.* ACF/CS/PLEN?ENDRINKS/16 Final. Brussels, Belgium: European Commission, Health & Consumer Protection Directorate-General, Scientific Committee on Food. http://ec.europa.eu/food/fs/sc/scf/out169_en.pdf (accessed November 26, 2013).

Somogyi, L. P. 2010. *Caffeine intake in the U.S. population.* http://www.fda.gov/downloads/AboutFDA/CentersOffices/OfficeofFoods/CFSAN/CFSANFOIAElectronicReadingRoom/UCM333191.pdf (accessed January 8, 2014).

Trabulo, D., S. Marques, and E. Pedroso. 2011. Caffeinated energy drink intoxication. *BMJ Case Reports* 2011 (February 2). doi:10.1136/bcr.09.2010.3322.

van Dam, R. M., W. J. Pasman, and P. Verheof. 2004. Effects of coffee consumption on fasting blood glucose and insuling concentrations: Randomized controlled trials in healthy volunteers. *Diabetes Care* 27(12):2990–2992.

Wedick, N. M., A. M. Brennan, Q. Sun, F. B. Hu, C. S. Mantzoros, and R. M. van Dam. 2011. Effects of caffeinated and decaffeinated coffee on biological risk factors for type 2 diabetes: A randomized controlled trial. *Nutrition Journal* 10:93.

4

Exploring Safe Caffeine Exposure Levels for Vulnerable Populations

Although the challenge of gaining a better scientific understanding of potentially vulnerable populations was addressed throughout the workshop in different contexts, the Day 2, Session 3, panel was designed to focus specifically on vulnerable populations. This chapter summarizes that panel. Moderator Mark Feeley, M.Sc., Health Canada, Ottawa, Ontario, asked the panelists to consider three key questions: (1) Are there specific vulnerable subpopulations that can be defined? (2) Are there additional variables beyond individual caffeine sensitivity that should be considered in these subpopulations as a means to help identify caffeine sensitivity? (3) What are the most relevant end points for defining a sensitive population? Many of the panelists' remarks and subsequent discussion revolved around currently established safe levels and the evidence underlying those levels. Box 4-1 describes key messages from the speakers.

BOX 4-1
Key Points Made by Individual Speakers

As noted by Mark Feeley, on the basis of an extensive scientific evaluation conducted about 10 years ago, Health Canada recommended that individuals consume no more than 400 mg of caffeine daily. Since then, Health Canada has identified two potentially vulnerable subpopulations, women of reproductive age and children, and has further recommended that children consume no more than 2.5 mg of caffeine per kilogram body weight per day and that women of reproductive age consume no more than 300 mg a day. Feeley discussed these standards, noting that the challenge with caffeine-containing energy drinks is similar to what the U.S. Food and Drug Administration is facing.

Christina Chambers said that several studies have indicated an increased risk for spontaneous abortion with caffeine consumption in pregnant women, prompting the American College of Obstetrics and Gynecology to recommend that pregnant women restrict their intake to less than 200 mg per day. Chambers described these studies and other evidence of health effects in pregnant women and made a call for better and more continuous measures of caffeine exposure during pregnancy.

Steven Lipshultz described the efforts of a working group in South Florida that was formed in 2007–2008 to see whether the safety signals being observed in children who had consumed caffeinated energy drinks were of concern. He identified children and children with underlying cardiac conditions as two potentially vulnerable populations. He encouraged banning the sale of caffeinated energy drinks to children and teenagers until and unless their safety can be demonstrated through scientific research.

HEALTH CANADA'S APPROACH

Introductory Remarks by Mark Feeley, M.Sc., Health Canada

Health Canada's position on caffeine is not much different from the Food and Drug Administration (FDA) position, according to Mark Feeley. When added directly to a food, caffeine is regulated as a food additive, requiring an application to Health Canada and a standard safety assessment. Approvals are granted on a case-by-case basis. Initially, the use of caffeine as a food additive in Canada was restricted to cola-type beverages; in the mid-2000s it was expanded to include all carbonated soft drinks. So today, theoretically, adding caffeine to a food for sale in Canada is restricted to carbonated soft drinks. Regulations regarding energy drinks are currently in flux, with most energy drinks on the market in the United States also having market access in Canada with some slight modifications to their composition.

About 10 years ago, Health Canada undertook a relatively extensive scientific evaluation of caffeine, from which it determined that a level of up to 400 mg of caffeine on a daily basis would likely not be associated with any adverse health effects in the general population. Subsequent to that review, Health Canada identified two potentially vulnerable subpopulations: women of reproductive age and children.

Women of reproductive age were identified as a potentially vulnerable group on the basis of the literature. Most studies examined by Health Canada focused on either reproductive or developmental outcomes and were based on coffee consumption as a surrogate for caffeine exposure. According to Feeley, most of the studies examined by Health Canada are described in an Oak Ridge National Laboratory (ORNL) report (2011), a very extensive evaluation that was conducted at the request of the FDA and whose conclusions were consistent with those of Health Canada. The studies did not show a clear cause-effect relationship between caffeine consumption and adverse health effects, with about 20 percent showing no effect, but they did show associations between caffeine consumption and some fertility indices. Health Canada decided that it would be prudent to suggest limiting caffeine intake among women of reproductive age to not more than 300 mg per day.

For children, the majority of evidence reviewed by Health Canada focused on children between 7 and 12 years of age. Most studies involved children being brought into a clinical setting and provided with defined caffeine doses through beverage exposure and with doses ranging from 2.5 to 10 mg per kg of body weight per day. Again, Feeley referred workshop participants to the ORNL (2011) review for what he described as an "elegant compilation" of the evidence. Beneficial effects were observed in terms of task, motor activity, attention, and other outcomes. But negative effects were observed as well. The one negative effect that was observed both consistently and at the lowest dose level was anxiety (i.e., both subjective and objective measurements of anxiety). On the basis of that research, although limited, Health Canada decided that it would be prudent to limit caffeine intake among children up to the age of 12 to no more than 2.5 mg per kg of body weight per day.

Feeley observed that median intakes in these subpopulations do not come close to these recommended maximum values. Only above the 90th percentile in either subpopulation have researchers observed individuals exceeding the recommended maximum levels. Health Canada is currently exploring options for product labeling and consumer education as ways to control the intakes of caffeine below the recommended daily intakes.

SAFE CAFFEINE EXPOSURE LEVELS IN VULNERABLE POPULATIONS: PREGNANT WOMEN AND INFANTS

Presented by Christina Chambers, Ph.D., M.P.H.,
University of California, San Diego

Christina Chambers listed several end points of interest with any exposure during pregnancy (i.e., not just caffeine): increased risk of spontaneous abortion or spontaneous pregnancy loss, typically defined as loss prior to 20 weeks' gestation; increased risk for major congenital anomalies; intrauterine growth restriction; and preterm birth. End points of interest with exposure to caffeine in infants, which occurs primarily through lactation, include increased risk for central nervous system effects, such as irritability and sleeplessness, and infant growth problems.

Chambers said that researchers who study caffeine exposure in pregnant women are challenged by several measurement and design issues, including limited capability to ethically conduct randomized clinical trials. Observational studies themselves are limited by their frequent reliance on maternal report of major sources of caffeine, some of which the mother may not be aware of, and misclassification of exposure in terms of timing and dose. Mothers are often being asked months or years after pregnancy to recall specific times that they consumed caffeine-containing products and doses of caffeine consumed. Observational studies that incorporate biomarker assessment (i.e., biomarkers of exposure) typically do so only at select time points and do not necessarily reflect exposure over time. Observational studies can also be challenged by either bias issues or confounding comorbidities such as depression or other maternal psychiatric disorders, autoimmune diseases, maternal diet (i.e., it may be different in high versus low caffeine consumers), and maternal body mass index. Also, there may be coexposures associated with higher caffeine intake, such as alcohol and tobacco.

Finally, an important problem, especially with studying spontaneous abortion, is the change in usual caffeine consumption because of the symptoms of pregnancy. More than half of pregnant women experience nausea and vomiting, which, in turn, may lead to reduced caffeine consumption. But nausea and vomiting are also highly protective against spontaneous abortion, potentially confounding any found association between caffeine consumption and spontaneous abortion. For this and other reasons, according to Chambers, spontaneous abortion is one of the most difficult pregnancy outcomes to study appropriately.

The challenge to studying spontaneous abortion is compounded by the fact that although spontaneous abortion is an extremely common event, occurring in 60 percent or more of pregnancies, is usually not clinically recognized. Also, because it may be more socially acceptable or preferable for a mother to report that she had a spontaneous abortion than a medically induced abortion, spontaneous abortion is sometimes misclassified. Finally, although most spontaneous abortions are believed to be caused by chromosome aberrations, not environmental exposure, many known environmental risk factors that might be associated with high caffeine exposure, such as the quantity and frequency of tobacco use, are poorly measured.

Despite these challenges, said Chambers, several studies have suggested increased risk for spontaneous abortion with caffeine consumption, particularly with higher doses. She described one study that drew attention in the past several years by Weng et al. (2008). The study focused on 1,063 women enrolled in the Kaiser health care plan in northern California. The women, all of whom tested positive for pregnancy, were interviewed subsequent to their pregnancy tests, sometime in the first 15 to 16 weeks of gestation, at a median age of 10 weeks of gestation. They were asked about previous caffeine consumption up to that time. Chambers noted that some women had already experienced a spontaneous abortion at the time of the interview and that those women were being interviewed retrospectively. The researchers reported a hazard ratio of 1.42 for a spontaneous abortion among women who consumed, on average, less than 200 mg of caffeine per day. That value, she said, was not statistically significant. For women who consumed 200 mg or more per day, the hazard ratio rose to 2.23, with a lower bound to the confidence interval of 1.34. Accounting for nausea and vomiting, the researchers concluded that doses of 200 mg or more per day were associated with an increased risk, about a doubling of risk, for spontaneous abortion.

A conflicting study was published the same year. Savitz et al. (2008) collected data on caffeine consumption by interviewing 2,407 women enrolled in a cohort either prior to pregnancy or during early pregnancy. The researchers reported that caffeine consumption was unrelated to an increased risk of spontaneous abortion if the event occurred after data collection on caffeine, that is, among women who were interviewed prior to knowing they were going to have spontaneous abortions. Among women who were interviewed after already experiencing spontaneous abortions, the researchers found an association. They concluded that there was no evidence of an increased risk for spontaneous abortion with caffeine consumption at any level within the range of the study and that the association found among women who had already experienced spontaneous abortions was a spurious association resulting from recall bias.

Despite these conflicting results, concern for risk of spontaneous abortion led the American College of Obstetrics and Gynecology to issue guidelines recommending that pregnant women restrict their caffeine intake to less than 200 mg per day.

Evidence for congenital anomalies as a potential adverse health effect associated with caffeine consumption during pregnancy has been somewhat unremarkable, according to Chambers. A number of recent studies have examined increased risk relative to a variety of specific defects that might be expected if caffeine were a teratogen. Most recently, the National Birth Defects Prevention Study,[1] a Centers for Disease Control and Prevention (CDC) multicenter study, which now has sufficient numbers of specific birth defects to provide adequate statistical power, has yielded variable and not very compelling results. There has been little evidence of a dose–response relationship. In addition, animal models at doses relevant to human exposure have not been concerning. In sum, in Chambers' opinion, the evidence is not compelling enough to suggest that there is an increased risk for any specific pattern of congenital anomalies in humans with caffeine consumption in the range that women would typically consume.

Nor have researchers found a consistent association between caffeine consumption during pregnancy and various measures of fetal growth, including increased risk for growth, small for gestational age, and low birth weight. Chambers described a 2008 study on small for gestational age and low birth weight among 2,635 women that showed little evidence of a dose relation in various dosing ranges (all greater than 100 mg per day) compared to women who consumed less than 100 mg per day. Odds ratios ranged from 1.2 to 1.5, with two showing borderline statistical significance, but again, with no evidence of a dose–response relationship with increasing levels of consumption (CARE Study Group, 2008). Likewise, even studies showing positive associations have suggested relatively small effects in terms of magnitude, too small to be clinically significant.

Finally, there have been a couple of noteworthy studies on preterm birth. Bech et al. (2007) conducted a randomized trial of caffeine reduction with two groups of pregnant women: one group received caffeinated coffee, the other decaffeinated coffee. Among the 1,207 women, the researchers found no effect of caffeine consumption on length of gestation at an average intake of 182 mg per day. Clausson et al. (2002) reported no association among 873 pregnant women between caffeine consumption at any level and preterm birth.

Among all these various studies of pregnant women, few have incorporated urine blood or core blood markers of exposure. In those studies that have included biomarkers, the biomarkers appear to be correlated with maternal report. According to Chambers, caffeine does not seem to carry the same stigma that alcohol and perhaps tobacco consumption do.

---

[1] Available at http://www.nbdps.org/index.html (accessed December 25, 2013).

Still, Chambers cautioned that most studies involve spot measures, which may not reflect individual genetic variability or changes over the course of pregnancy. A few studies have been conducted on the relation between polymorphisms for metabolizing enzymes and adverse health outcomes to see whether rapid metabolizers are at different risks, but the results have been conflicting.

With respect to infant exposure through caffeine in breast milk, there have been anecdotal individual case reports or small case series of fussiness, jitteriness, and poor sleep patterns among infants born to mothers who consume the equivalent of 10 or more cups of coffee daily. As with many agents in infants being breastfed, the effects can be amplified in preterm or very young infants (until the age of about 4 to 5 months) because they metabolize caffeine more slowly and may attain similar levels to their mothers. One study from Costa Rica suggested that coffee intake of more than 450 ml caffeine daily may decrease breast milk iron concentrations (Munoz et al., 1988).

Data Gaps

To conclude, Chambers identified several data gaps:

- Better and more continuous measures of exposure at specific time points and at repeated time points over pregnancy. Such data would help researchers to tease apart real risks and determine whether there is a peak exposure effect or critical time of exposure.
- Data that would help determine whether there are any neurobehavioral effects of high dose exposure that are independent of the effects of coexposure, such as alcohol and tobacco.
- Data on the dose of exposure and potential effects during the 5- to 6-week period prior to a woman realizing that she is pregnant. This is an important piece of information, in Chambers's opinion, because more than half of all pregnant women do not plan their pregnancies. So, for example, among women who are not aware that they are pregnant, what is the pattern of energy drink consumption? What is the pattern of alcohol consumption? Are women who consume energy drinks binge drinking? Is high caffeine consumption in an unrecognized pregnancy associated with poor dietary habits? Is high caffeine consumption in an unrecognized pregnancy associated with lack of use of folic acid supplements, which in turn may lead to an increased risk of birth defects?

- Data in humans on the effects of other ingredients in caffeinated energy drinks and other products.

RISK OF ADVERSE EFFECTS OF CAFFEINE AND CAFFEINATED PRODUCTS IN CHILDREN AND OTHER VULNERABLE GROUPS

Presented by Steven E. Lipshultz, M.D., University of Miami

In 2007, physicians in south Florida were seeing health effects in children that seemed to be temporally related to the use of caffeinated energy drinks. Steven Lipshultz described how he and his colleagues formed a working group to determine whether those safety signals were of concern.

The group interviewed the south Florida poison control center database. In 2007, across the state of Florida, 39 persons, aged 2 to 20 years, were being tracked for health concerns associated with caffeine consumption. In 2008, 125 persons aged 2 to 20 years were being tracked. Those cases were only for general caffeine toxicity because at the time there was no reporting mechanism in the United States for caffeine toxicity related to energy drink consumption.

Next, the group interviewed the National Poison Control Center database, again focusing on caffeine. They reported their results in *Pediatrics* (Seifert et al., 2011). They found that children from infants to age 19 years accounted for 46 percent of all calls reporting caffeine toxicity in 2007. About 10 percent of these cases had moderately severe symptoms that often required treatment. There were deaths in all years examined (2006–2008).

The working group, Lipshultz noted, eventually became aware that the Substance Abuse and Mental Health Services Administration was collecting data on U.S. emergency department visits involving caffeinated energy drink consumption in patients 12 years old and older. Those data, which were published in a 2011 DAWN report (SAMHSA, 2013), suggested that such visits increased exponentially between 2005 and 2011 (see Figure 4-1).

He also noted that the working group sought data from outside the United States as well. Caffeinated energy drink toxicity has been tracked elsewhere, notably in Australia, Germany, Ireland, and New Zealand. The German Federal Institute for Risk Assessment assessed caffeinated energy drink toxicity from 2002 to 2008 and reported several serious outcomes: liver damage, kidney failure, respiratory disorders, agitation, seizures, psychotic conditions, rhabdomyolysis, tachycardia, cardiac arrhythmias, hypertension, heart failure, and death. From 1999 through 2005, Ireland's poison center reported seventeen adverse events associated with energy drinks, including confusion, tachycardia, and seizures and two deaths. Furthermore, Lipshultz said, from 2005 to 2009, the New Zealand poison center reported 20 energy drink– or energy shot–related adverse events, including vomiting, nausea, abdominal pain, jitteriness, racing heart, agitation, and myocardial infarction. Between 2004 and 2010, the New South Wales Australian Poison Information Center reported increases in both recreational ingestions and accidental pediatric ingestions of caffeinated energy drinks (Gunja and Brown, 2012; see Figure 4-2).

This information led the group to discuss the need to track caffeinated energy drink toxicity with the U.S. National Poison Data System (NPDS). Lipshultz and his colleagues were pleased to learn that the NPDS had recognized the same need. Data from the first year of reporting (from October 1, 2010, through September 30, 2011) were published in *Clinical Toxicology* (Seifert et al., 2013). During that period, there were 1,480 cases of nonalcoholic caffeinated energy drink toxicity, half of which involved children younger than 6 years old. Specifically, 51 percent involved children 0 to 5 years old; 11 percent, children 6 to 12 years old; 18 percent, teenagers 13 to 19 years old; and 21 percent, adults 20 years and older. Children under the age of 6 years also had the highest proportion of unintentional exposures to nonalcoholic energy drinks (76 percent), and teenagers between 13 and 19 years had the highest proportion of intentional exposures (49 percent).

In 2012, the New Zealand Food Safety Authority compared the effects of exposure to caffeine from energy drinks or energy shots to background dietary exposure from naturally occurring caffeine in foods and beverages and in cola-type soft drinks (Thompson and Schiess, 2010). They found that 68 percent of children and 42 percent of teenagers exceeded the adverse-effect level of 3 mg caffeine per kg body weight after consuming one retail unit of energy drink or energy shot beyond their baseline dietary exposure (Thompson and Schiess, 2010; Seifert et al., 2011).

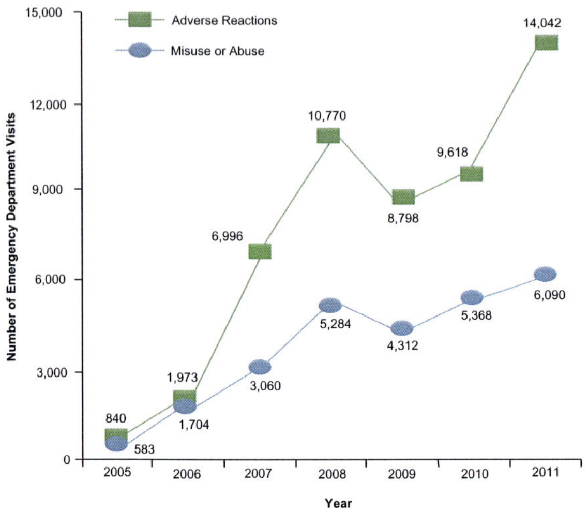

FIGURE 4-1 U.S. emergency department visits involving caffeinated energy drinks in patients age 12 years and older, 2005–2011.
NOTE: An adverse reaction is defined as an adverse reaction or side effect to the use of energy drinks as documented in the chart; misuse or abuse is broadly defined to include all visits associated with inappropriate use of energy drinks.
SOURCE: SAMHSA, 2013. Presented to the Planning Committee for a Workshop on Potential Health Hazards Associated with Consumption of Caffeine in Food and Dietary Supplements on August 5, 2013.

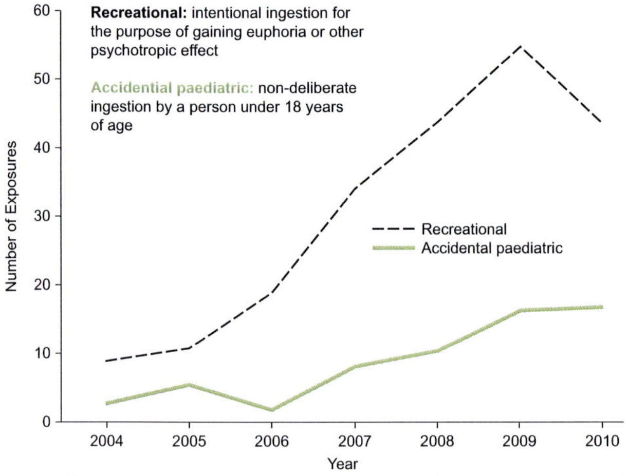

FIGURE 4-2 Calls regarding the intentional or accidental consumption of energy drinks to individual New South Wales, Australia, poison control centers, 2004–2010.
SOURCE: Gunja and Brown, 2012.

Children with Underlying Cardiac Disease as a Potentially Vulnerable Population

Lipshultz elaborated on the lack of screening in U.S. children for underlying heart disease and other susceptibilities. In his experience, many children are not aware of their underlying cardiac conditions. Sometimes the first event is terminal, and the underlying cardiac disease is identified only at autopsy.

The American College of Cardiology recommends restricting activities that increase adrenergic stimulation for groups at risk of sudden cardiac death. According to Lipshultz, some of the risks are the same as those associated with sudden death from exposure to caffeinated energy drinks, specifically hypertrophic cardiomyopathy and long QT syndrome. Dufendach et al. (2012) reported on a 13-year-old girl with no known history of cardiac disease who was taken to the emergency department. She had palpitations, chest pain, shakiness, and dizziness and had recently consumed a 16-ounce can of an energy drink containing 160 mg of caffeine (amounting to 4.1 mg per kg of body weight). After extensive testing, doctors diagnosed long QT syndrome.

Lipshultz noted that other regulatory groups already recognize risk groups for stimulants in addition to caffeine, such as those at risk from amphetamines used to treat attention deficit hyperactivity disorder (ADHD). In February 2005, Health Canada suspended the use of the amphetamine Adderall XR as a result of concerns about an increased risk of sudden cardiac death. In August of the same year, they reinstated the product but with revised labeling that identified rare heart-related side effects. In May 2006, the FDA directed manufacturers to strengthen the warning section of their labeling for Adderall XR by listing potentially serious cardiovascular adverse events.

For Lipshultz, it is not clear how best to balance the need to provide necessary medications to children with the need to protect children who have underlying heart disease. The south Florida working group asked itself whether any of its own specialists would recommend that children on hypertensive therapy for high blood pressure or children on anticonvulsant therapy for seizures not consume caffeine. These specialists believed that children on either type of therapy should probably be advised not to consume caffeine from any source.

High blood pressure, Lipshultz said, occurs in 3 to 5 percent of children in the United States, with 2.5 percent of NPDS calls for caffeinated energy drink consumption toxicity in the 2000–2013 period related to hypertension. Over the same period, 24 percent of reported caffeinated energy drink poisonings involved seizures. Caffeinated energy drinks may interfere with anticonvulsant therapy and lower the threshold for seizures. The situation is the same for children with syncopal disorders. Most physicians would advise children with syncopal disorders to not consume caffeine.

Similarly, about 10 percent of U.S. children have a diagnosis of ADHD. About 70 percent of these children are treated with prescription therapy, most commonly with stimulants. Most physicians would advise patients on stimulant therapy not to consume an additional stimulant. Lipshultz mentioned caloric intake and diabetes as another area of concern, with caffeine potentially exacerbating the adverse health outcomes associated with these conditions. In addition, among adolescents with eating disorders, caffeine can potentially lead to adverse health outcomes.

For children with underlying heart disease, any stimulant is of concern, whether it be a prescription medication or a caffeinated energy drink. Unfortunately, noted Lipshultz, routine physical exams for high school athletes do not identify everyone at risk for sudden cardiac death, nor are children in the United States routinely examined with electrocardiography or echocardiography.

Various national organizations and individuals have put forth recommendations for the use of energy drinks among children, including the American Academy of Pediatrics, perhaps the largest pediatric organization in the world. In 2013, the American Medical Association voted that marketing energy drinks to children and adolescents less than 18 years old should be suspended. According to Lipshultz, these various educational campaigns, as well as the banning of the sale of alcohol-containing energy drinks by the FDA, appear to be associated with decreasing calls to poison centers for energy drink consumption (see Figure 4-3).

In his conclusion, Lipshultz reiterated that not only do caffeine-containing energy drinks have no therapeutic or nutritional benefit for children less than 18 years of age, but also all available databases suggest that certain subgroups may experience serious adverse events after consuming these drinks. Are there safety signals? "There are absolute safety signals," Lipshultz said. "It's consistent in every study that we can get our hands on." He identified two probable vulnerable populations: children and children with underlying disease. Lipshultz said that until research establishes the children's safety, "as a pediatrician, as somebody who's run one of the largest children's hospitals for a decade, it is part of my responsibility to protect children when I see safety signals until I really know there's a therapeutic benefit or at least no increased risk."

PANELIST DISCUSSION WITH THE AUDIENCE

Lipshultz clarified that no data indicate any specific safety threshold in suspected highly vulnerable populations, such as children with underlying cardiac or other conditions. Until such data become available and without any data to suggest that there is a therapeutic advantage to consuming caffeine-containing energy drinks, he reiterated his recommendation that children with underlying cardiac conditions not consume such products.

The National Poison Data System: An Imperfect System

An audience member commented on Dr. Lipshultz's observation that 51 percent of all reported energy drink poisonings involved children

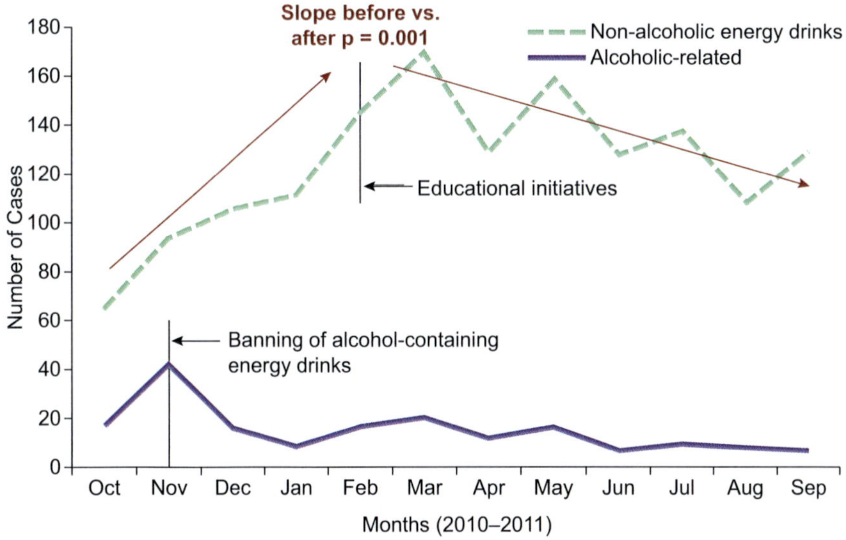

FIGURE 4-3 Poison center energy drink calls over time, 2010–2011.
NOTE: Calls made before and after the FDA ban on the sale of alcohol-containing energy drinks and before and after the initiation of public education campaigns about the risks of caffeine-containing energy drinks.
SOURCE: Seifert et al., 2013.

younger than 6 years of age. The commenter observed that most of the 717 cases involving children under age 6 are trivial cases in which a parent calls and the poison center specialist learns, for example, that the child came into contact with an energy drink by touching a can to their mouths. On the basis of his own calculations, the commenter concluded that 82 percent of the 717 cases were "no effect" cases. The commenter remarked on the difference between a "poisoning" and an "exposure" as reported in the NPDS database.

Lipshultz replied that such a calculation is possible because those data are now available and that the NPDS is operating under full disclosure. He noted that these data were initial first-year data and acknowledged that such limited data can be overinterpreted. Thus, he and his colleagues are in the process of analyzing the first 3 years of data. As part of that analysis, they are comparing caffeine exposures associated with energy drinks to caffeine exposures associated with other products. One of the frustrations for him concerning NPDS data is the low level of follow-up to verify facts and to ascertain outcomes. He reiterated, "It's a very imperfect system."

With respect to the word "poisoning," he noted that it is a definitional term. Because the calls are made to poison centers, they are logged as "poisonings."

For Lipshultz, the key point is that, regardless of which database one examines, whether in Australia, Germany, Ireland, New Zealand, the United States, or elsewhere, one observes very similar findings. He reiterated, "There's not one perfect way to ascertain adverse effects of energy-drink consumption when cases are not being tracked in a systematic way." He cautioned against relying on consumption data only, without examining NPDS health-consequence data. Consumption data suggest no consumption among young children, yet real toxicities are being observed in such children worldwide. In fact, that apparent discrepancy may indicate an even more vulnerable population than children, that is, children with underlying medical conditions. Lipshultz referred to earlier presentations on consumption data analyzed by two separate groups and the challenges those groups are having with respect to quantifying consumption.

In Lipshultz's opinion, safety signals are being observed. Calls are being received by a variety of people that relate to temporal associations with these products. The next step is to verify those signals at "the next level of higher-quality science."

When asked about the need for a national registry to track adverse events associated with caffeinated energy drink consumption or the need for mandated reporting of such events, Lipshultz replied that the NPDS is an imperfect system but that it is the best means currently available for tracking such events in any "semi-systematic" way. That said, he supports efforts to more carefully examine safety issues related to caffeinated energy drink consumption.

Following Lipschultz's presentation, audience members were invited to ask questions of the panelists. This section summarizes the discussion that took place. Most of the questions revolved around how some of the data presented are being interpreted and the gaps in data.

Questions About Data on Pregnant Women as a Vulnerable Population

Chambers was asked whether there is any evidence for the mutagenicity of caffeine. She replied that there is none.

In response to a question about monotonic linear dose responses, Chambers clarified that the lack of such a response for small for gestational age does not necessarily suggest that there is no effect. It could be a nonlinear relationship. Smoking, for example, has an effect on craniosynostosis at low and moderate doses but not at high doses. Or it could be that there is an effect but that the effect is impacted by other phenomena.

Finally, Chambers was asked about compliancy among pregnant women with respect to recommendations for reduced caffeine consumption. The commenter referred to a study showing that women who met diagnostic criteria for caffeine dependence were less likely to reduce caffeine consumption below the Health Canada recommended 300 mg daily. Although not familiar with any data on compliance, Chambers suspected that most pregnant women are not compliant. She wonders whether pregnant women who are addicted to caffeine and to other substances are "particularly recalcitrant" to reducing their caffeine consumption. "That's an important question," she said. She also pointed to the need to examine caffeine withdrawal during pregnancy. Some of the symptoms of withdrawal are similar to those of pregnancy. As far as she knows, no one has examined that yet.

REFERENCES

Bech, B. H., C. Obel, T. Brink Henrickson, and J. Olsen. 2007. Effect of reducing caffeine intake on birth weight and length of gestation: Randomised controlled trial. *British Medical Journal.* doi:10.1136/bmj.39062.520648.BE.

CARE Study Group. 2008. Maternal caffeine intake during pregnancy and risk of fetal growth restriction: A large prospective observational study. *British Medical Journal* 337:a2332. doi:10.1136/bmj.a2332.

Clausson, B., F. Granath, A. Ekbom, S. Lundgren, A. Nordmark, and L. B. Signorello. 2002. *American Journal of Epidemiology* 155(5):429–436.

Dufendach, K. A., J. M. Horner, B. C. Cannon, and M. J. Ackerman. 2012. Congenital type 1 long QT syndrome unmasked by a highly caffeinated energy drink. *Heart Rhythm* 9:285–288.

Gunja, N., and J. A. Brown. 2012. Energy drinks: Health risks and toxicity. *Medical Journal of Australia* 196:46–49.

Munoz, L. M., B. Lonnerdale, C. L. Keen, and K. G. Dewey. 1988. Coffee consumption as a factor in iron deficiency anemia among pregnant women and their infants in Costa Rica. *American Journal of Clinical Nutrition* 48:645–651.

ORNL (Oak Ridge National Laboratory). 2011. *Adverse health effects of caffeine: Review and analysis of recent human and animal research.* http://iom.edu/~/media/Files/Activity%20Files/Nutrition/PotentialEffectsof Caffeine/caffeineORNLreport.pdf (accessed February 10, 2014).

SAMHSA (Substance Abuse and Mental Health Services Administration). 2013. *Drug Abuse Warning Network (DAWN) report: Update on emergency department visits involving energy drinks: A continuing public health concern.* http://www.samhsa.gov/data/2k13/DAWN126/sr126-energy-drinks-use.pdf (accessed November 25, 2013).

Savitz, D. A., R. L. Chan, A. H. Herring, P. P. Howards, and K. E. Hartmann. 2008. Caffeine and miscarriage risk. *Epidemiology* 19:55–62.

Seifert, S. M., J. L. Schaechter, E. R. Hershorin, and S. E. Lipshultz. 2011. Health effects of energy drinks on children, adolescents, and young adults. *Pediatrics* 127:511–528.

Seifert, S. M., S. A. Seifert, J. L. Schaechter, A. C. Bronstein, B. E. Benson, E. R. Hershorin, K. L. Arheart, V. I. Franco, and S. E. Lipshultz. 2013. An analysis of energy-drink toxicity in the National Poison Data System. *Clinical Toxicology* 51:566–574.

Thompson, B., and S. Schiess. 2010. *Risk profile: Caffeine in energy drinks and energy shots.* Report prepared for New Zealand Food Safety Authority under project CFS/09/04. Christchurch, New Zealand: Institute of Environmental Science and Research Limited.

Weng, X., R. Odouli, and D. K. Li. 2008. Maternal caffeine consumption during pregnancy and the risk of miscarriage: A prospective cohort study. *American Journal of Obstetrics and Gynecology* 198:279.e1–279.e8.

5

Caffeine Effects on the Cardiovascular System

Much of the concern about caffeinated food and beverages and their potential health effects in vulnerable populations stems from several recent sudden cardiac deaths in adolescents being attributed to consumption of caffeinated energy drinks. However, during the workshop, some experts questioned the causal nature of the relationship. Others warned that, at the very least, the deaths are an early safety signal that warrants further investigation. Some workshop participants who spoke urged that until such investigation demonstrates the safety of caffeinated energy drinks in children, adolescents, pregnant women, caffeine-sensitive individuals, and other vulnerable populations, it would be prudent to restrict their use. In the Day 1, Session 3, panel, moderated by Stephen R. Daniels, M.D., Ph.D., Department of Pediatrics, University of Colorado School of Medicine, Denver, panelists explored the current state of the science on the effects of caffeine on the cardiovascular system. Box 5-1 describes the key points made by each speaker.

VASCULAR EFFECTS OF CAFFEINE

Presented by John P. Higgins, M.D., M.B.A., University of Texas Medical School

Endothelial cell function (ECF) serves an important role in mediating the vascular effects of caffeine exposure, according to John Higgins. He described normal[1] and abnormal[2] ECF and potential implications of abnormal ECF for cardiac health; explained how caffeine in individuals at rest appears to improve ECF but that caffeine in individuals during exercise appears to reduce ECF; and presented data suggesting that energy drinks in individuals at rest also reduce ECF.

Endothelial Cell Function

Endothelial cells form the inner lining of blood vessels and serve both basal and inducible metabolic and synthetic functions (Sumpio et

BOX 5-1
Key Points Made by Individual Speakers

John Higgins discussed data showing that endothelial cell function mediates the vascular effects of caffeine exposure, with implications for cardiac health. Caffeine in an individual at rest appears to improve endothelial cell function. In combination with exercise, however, caffeine appears to decrease endothelial cell function. Energy drinks in individuals at rest also decreases endothelial cell function. Higgins emphasized the need for more research on the effects of caffeine, exercise, and energy drinks on endothelial cell function, especially among younger individuals.

Jeffrey Goldberger noted that physicians have long recommended reducing caffeine consumption in patients complaining of heart palpitations. Goldberger explored available evidence on the effects of caffeine on the risk of arrhythmia. He concluded that although some data indicate dose-dependent effects on some cardiac parameters, including heart rate and blood pressure, prevailing evidence suggests no effect on arrhythmia. In his opinion, clinical advice to limit caffeine consumption is based primarily on anecdote and folklore, though some people may have individual sensitivity to caffeine.

Genetic variation in response to caffeine may explain some of the mixed results being reported for various cardiovascular system functions, according to Ahmed El-Sohemy. El-Sohemy described evidence suggesting that variation in CYP1A2, a gene that encodes an important caffeine metabolism enzyme, likely plays a role. El-Sohemy emphasized the importance of both personalized and public health advice and urged identification of vulnerable genotypes.

Both Higgins and El-Sohemy suggested that caffeine may exert different effects when delivered in caffeinated energy drinks compared to coffee and other traditional modes of caffeine delivery.

[1]Normal endothelial function is characterized by vasodilatation, thromboresistance, and blood cell antiadhesion.

[2]Abnormal endothelial function is characterized by vasoconstriction of the arteries, procoagulant effects, and proadhesion of blood cells.

al., 2002). Among other multiple tasks, normal ECF serves an important role in regulating vascular tone (i.e., blood vessel tone), preventing thrombosis (i.e., the ability of blood to clot in the artery), and preventing arterial damage by acting as a barrier. Higgins described ECF as a "balancing act," with normal ECF being associated with vasodilatation (i.e., larger arteries), thromboresistance (i.e., thinner blood, which prevents blood clots), and antiadhesion. With respect to antiadhesion, Higgins compared normal ECF to the Teflon coating on a frying pan: when it is working well, things do not stick. The molecules that appear to be important for normal ECF are nitric oxide, prostaglandin I2, endothelium-derived hyperpolarizing factor, and bradykinin.

Abnormal ECF, on the other hand, manifests as vasoconstriction (i.e., smaller arteries), procoagulant effects (i.e., blood clot), and proadhesion, said Higgins. Molecules that appear to play an important role in abnormal ECF include renin, angiotensin, endothelin 1, and others.

Abnormal ECF is important in both the short term and the long term. In the short term, during stress or certain exposures—for example, in cold temperatures or during exposure to cigarette smoke or cocaine—abnormal ECF impairs the ability of arteries to dilate normally and potentially could result in a supply-demand imbalance, that is, with the heart beating harder and needing more blood flow while at the same time not being able to open up the arteries to improve blood flow. This supply-demand imbalance could in the short term lead to ischemia and possibly cardiac arrhythmia. In the long term, abnormal ECF can lead to hypertension, atherosclerosis, cardiovascular disease, coronary disease, and peripheral artery disease.

Improving ECF is a desirable goal, with many ways to do so, including exercise, smoking cessation, certain antioxidants (e.g., vitamin C, flavonoids in dark chocolate), cholesterol-lowering statins, omega-3 fatty acids, glycemic control in diabetes, L-arginine (i.e., a precursor to nitric oxide), and angiotensin-converting enzyme inhibitors and angiotensin-receptor blockers (Widlansky et al., 2003; Lee et al., 2012).

Caffeine in Individuals at Rest Improves ECF

Caffeine in individuals at rest is believed to improve ECF by increasing intracellular calcium, which in turn stimulates expression of endothelial nitric oxide synthase, which itself stimulates the endothelial cells to produce nitric oxide. The nitric oxide then diffuses to the vascular smooth muscle, which lies just underneath the endothelial cells, and results in vascular smooth muscle vasodilatation (Echeverri et al., 2010). Caffeine can also bind directly to the vascular smooth muscle cell receptors and, through similar mechanisms, cause vasodilatation (Echeverri et al., 2010).

Higgins described two in vivo[3] studies on the ECF effects of caffeine in individuals at rest (Higgins and Babu, 2013). The first study involved 40 individuals, 33 of whom were male, with an average age of 53 years, all of whom consumed 200 mg of caffeine and were tested 60 minutes later using flow-mediated dilatation of the brachial artery. The researchers found that resting flow-mediated dilatation increased 10 percent after caffeine ingestion ($p < 0.001$). The second study involved 10 individuals, all males, with an average age of 27, all of whom consumed 300 mg of caffeine and were tested 60 minutes later using a strain-gauge plethysmograph to measure forearm blood flow. The researchers also measured blood flow responses to acetylcholine, which is an endothelium-dependent vasodilator, and to sodium nitroprusside, which is an endothelium-independent vasodilator. They found that resting forearm blood flow was not affected by caffeine but that resting forearm blood flow response to acetylcholine increased by 25 percent ($p < 0.05$). According to Higgins, these latter results suggest that the endothelium is very important in the vasorelaxation effect of caffeine in individuals at rest.

Equally significant, in Higgins's opinion, caffeine blocks adenosine receptors, which are important in dilating coronary arteries to augment coronary blood flow during exercise (Echeverri et al., 2010). This finding is important, he explained, because adenosine receptors are present throughout circulation where, in most places, they vasodilate, that is, they make arteries larger and thereby increase blood flow. For example, in the coronary arteries, the adenosine 2a receptor results in vasodilation. In the aorta, the adenosine 2b receptor does. Caffeine competitively blocks those and all other adenosine receptors, resulting in a compensatory increase in adenosine by the body, which in turn stimulates circulating chemoreceptors and other receptors, leading to an increase in sympathetic tone, catecholamines, peripheral vascular resistance, and renin secretion. These effects manifest as increased blood pressure, with systolic blood pressure increasing by 7 mm and diastolic blood pressure by 3 mm 60 minutes after ingestion of 300 mg of caffeine.

---

[3]In vivo refers to experiments conducted in a living organism: plant, animal, or human.

Caffeine Plus Exercise Decreases ECF

As a sports cardiologist, Higgins is especially interested in ECF as measured by myocardial blood flow. He described results from three studies based on measurements of either myocardial perfusion by positron emission tomography or brachial artery ECF by flow-mediated dilation (Higgins and Babu, 2013). Flow-mediated dilation measurements are also an accepted surrogate for coronary artery ECF (i.e., how well the brachial arteries in the arms can dilate correlates with how well the coronary arteries can dilate).

Higgins described the first study, which involved 15 subjects, 5 of whom were male, with an average age of 58 years, all of whom received 200 mg of pure caffeine and were then tested 50 minutes later while bicycling. Positron emission tomography was used to measure myocardial perfusion. The researchers found that exercise-induced myocardial blood flow response decreased 14 percent after caffeine ingestion ($p < 0.05$). So caffeine ingestion followed by exercise on a bicycle reduced coronary blood flow. The second study involved 18 individuals, 11 of whom were male, with an average age of 27 years, all of whom received 200 mg of pure caffeine and were then tested 50 minutes later while bicycling. The researchers found that exercise-induced myocardial blood flow response decreased 22 percent after caffeine ingestion ($p < 0.01$). The third study involved 10 individuals, with an average age of 30, who were administered 360 mg of caffeine and their forearm blood flow measured at baseline and then again every 20 minutes during 55 minutes of bicycling. Forearm blood flow was measured using a venous plethysmographic exclusion technique with a wrist cuff method of flow-mediated dilatation. The researchers found that, with individuals at rest, caffeine had no effect on forearm blood flow. During exercise, however, caffeine attenuated the usual increase in forearm blood flow by 53 percent ($p < 0.05$). In sum, caffeine plus exercise appears to decrease blood flow.

Energy Drinks in Individuals at Rest Decrease ECF

Higgins expressed concern that children and teenagers can purchase caffeine-containing energy drinks in stores. He observed that it is not uncommon for today's youth to consume cans of energy drinks at soccer game half-times, instead of the cut-up oranges or bananas that he and his peers used to consume as children during their soccer games/school events. He is concerned because he and his colleagues have witnessed many emergency room visits by children and adolescents after having consumed energy drinks. He also mentioned the wrongful death lawsuit filed against an energy drink company in October 2012 and a March 2013 letter to the FDA commissioner asking the FDA to examine the case reports of sudden cardiac death associated with energy drink consumption.

With this concern in mind, Higgins described the results of two studies on energy drinks and ECF. First, Worthley et al. (2010) measured two types of ECF in 50 healthy volunteers, including 34 males, with an average age of 22 years. The researchers measured adenosine disphosphate–induced platelet aggregation and the reactive hyperemia index (i.e., how the artery is able to dilate) both before and 1 hour after the volunteers consumed a 250-ml can of sugar-free energy drink. They reported a significant ($p < 0.007$) 13.7 percent increase in platelet aggregation following energy drink consumption, compared to basically no change in the control, and a significant ($p < 0.05$) reduction in reactive hyperemia index, again compared to a nonsignificant difference from baseline in the control. Also, not unexpectedly, according to Higgins, the researchers reported an increase in blood pressure following the energy beverage consumption ($p < 0.05$).

The second study Higgins described was based on his own research at the University of Texas Health Science Center. The study, SHADE-ONE (**S**tudy of **H**eart Effects from **A**dults **D**rinking **E**nergy Beverages: **On E**ndothelial Function), was a pilot study involving Higgins himself (Higgins, 2013). Measurements were taken prior to Higgins consuming a 24-ounce energy drink and then 90 minutes after consumption. At rest, Higgins's artery dilated to 0.42 cm and then to 0.45 cm after he performed flow-mediated dilatation using the standard cuff occlusion method. Ninety minutes after he drank the 24-ounce energy drink, his artery dilated to 0.43 cm but then only to 0.44 cm with maximal flow-mediated dilatation.

As part of SHADE-ONE, Higgins also measured percent flow-mediated dilatation at 50 minutes as well as at baseline and 90 minutes and found that it decreased over time and was lowest at 90 minutes. According to Higgins, most people's caffeine levels peak between 45 and 60 minutes after consumption. He found it interesting that with this energy drink, which he noted has other important ingredients in addition to caffeine, the maximal effect was observed at 90 minutes. The finding suggests to Higgins that there may be something about energy drinks that makes them "different beasts" than coffee and other modes of caffeine delivery. For example, maybe there is something in them that affects the pharmacokinetics or dynamics of caffeine by interacting with the caffeine and thereby having more deleterious effects on ECF.

Conclusions About Vascular Effects of Caffeine

Higgins concluded that in healthy individuals aged 22 to 59 years who consume 200 to 300 mg of caffeine, indirect tests indicate improved ECF and vasodilation at rest. So adults consuming this much caffeine during activities of daily living are likely safe, provided they are not caffeine sensitive, pregnant, or taking medication that interacts with caffeine or do not have a medical condition that is worsened by caffeine. For those who consume caffeine immediately before or during exercise, however, there could be harmful results. It appears that caffeine may attenuate the normal physiological mechanisms that help increase myocardial blood flow that occur during the increased demand of exercise. Researchers know that caffeine blocks adenosine receptors, thus reducing the ability of the coronary arteries to improve their flow commensurate with the increased myocardial demand of exercise. This could perhaps result in supply-demand ischemia. In healthy individuals aged 21 to 71 years who consume 200 to 300 mg of caffeine and then perform aerobic exercise 1 hour later, indirect tests indicate reduced ECF as measured by reduced myocardial blood flow. Finally, in healthy individuals aged 20 to 47 years who consume energy drinks, indirect tests indicate reduced ECF at rest.

Higgins called for more research on the effects of caffeine and energy drinks on ECF and the mechanisms underlying those effects and for more research on the safety of high-dose caffeine and energy drinks in younger individuals, caffeine-naïve individuals, and individuals who exercise 1 to 2 hours after consumption. In the 6 cases that he was aware of in which deaths were associated with energy drink consumption, affected individuals were between 12 and 19 years of age. He identified that age group as a potentially vulnerable population.

CAFFEINE AND RISK OF ARRHYTHMIA

Presented by Jeffrey Goldberger, M.D., Northwestern University

A 1994 survey of several hundred physicians from Minnesota and Vermont found that 94 percent of those surveyed recommended reducing or stopping caffeine for patients complaining of palpitations (Hughes et al., 1988). Jeffrey Goldberger described the finding as "remarkable" and considered it his task for the workshop to examine whether the evidence supports that recommendation. In his experience, it is not often that 94 percent of physicians agree on something even when its benefits have been demonstrated in randomized clinical trials, such as the use of beta-blockers after myocardial infarction or anticoagulants for atrial fibrillation. It is difficult to get that kind of consensus and interesting to consider where it comes from.

There are many data sources on the effects of caffeine on arrhythmias, including case reports, animal studies, human physiologic studies, human small-case series, and human observational trials. The predominant focus of Goldberger's presentation was on human observational trials. He noted that most of the data comes from coffee-intake studies and emphasized the need to keep in mind, while reviewing these studies, the variation in the amount of caffeine in different coffee drinks.

There are also many end points to consider when evaluating the effects of caffeine on the heart, including physiologic surrogates (i.e., electrophysiological effects such as QRS duration, which is the time required to depolarize the ventricles), specific arrhythmias, and epidemiological outcomes. He focused on three types of specific arrhythmias: (1) atrial fibrillation, a common arrhythmia in middle-aged and older individuals; (2) premature ventricular complexes, which are extra beats that arise from the ventricles and are common at all ages and in people either with or without heart disease; and (3) arrhythmias that can lead to sudden cardiac death, which include ventricular fibrillation and very rapid ventricular tachycardia.

Animal Studies on the Effect of Caffeine on Cardiac Arrhythmias

Goldberger described two animal studies that he thought were especially interesting. First, Bellet et al. (1972) examined the effect of caffeine on ventricular fibrillation thresholds in dogs. The researchers measured the amount of energy required to induce ventricular fibrillation with shocks to the heart among both control dogs and dogs that had experienced myocardial infarctions. They found that having had a myocardial infarction reduced the ventricular fibrillation threshold. In both groups of dogs, the ventricular fibrillation threshold was reduced even further when caffeine was administered. Goldberger noted, however, that the caffeine dose used was 25 mg per kg, which would amount to about 1.75 gm in a 70-kg man, not a typical human dose. In a second animal study, Rashid et al. (2006) examined the effect of caffeine on the inducibility of atrial fibrillation. They found that caffeine actually decreased the window of vulnerability for atrial fibrillation. Goldberger remarked that he was unsure of the clinical implications of this finding but found the study interesting because it reflects the range of caffeine effects observed in animals in relation to cardiac arrhythmias.

Human Studies on the Effect of Caffeine on Arrhythmias and Other Cardiac End Points

Many health effects that are observed in association with caffeine exposure are those that occur on sympathetic excitation, according to Goldberger. Corti et al. (2002) examined the effect of coffee on sympathetic nerve activity in a placebo-controlled trial of 15 healthy volunteers (6 habitual and 9 nonhabitual coffee drinkers). A number of interventions were tested, including intravenous caffeine (250 mg) versus placebo and a triple espresso (which was designed to mimic the 250-mg intravenous treatment) versus a decaf triple espresso (nonhabitual coffee drinkers only). The researchers reported a sustained increase in caffeine levels in the intravenous caffeine group and, not surprisingly in Goldberger's opinion, a small increase in blood pressure and a drop in heart rate. Sympathetic nerve activity, as measured by a number of different techniques, also increased. The placebo group showed no change over time. With coffee drinking, there was no difference between habitual versus nonhabitual coffee drinkers with respect to sympathetic nerve activity or caffeine levels. A striking finding, in Goldberger's opinion, was that decaf administered to nonhabitual users increased blood pressure and sympathetic nerve activity. Habitual users showed no increase in blood pressure.

In another study, Jackman et al. (1996) examined caffeine effects on catecholamines in 14 athletes during intense exercise. The researchers orally administered 6 mg of caffeine per kg 1 hour before exercise. The exercise protocol involved cycling at 2 minutes at a power required to achieve maximum oxygen uptake, resting for minutes, cycling again at the same power for 2 minutes, resting for 6, and then cycling at the same power to exhaustion. They found a slight increase in exercise endurance and significantly higher plasma epinephrine levels at peak exercise in the caffeine group. In Goldberger's opinion, the findings serve as evidence of sympathoexcitation.

In one of the first studies on caffeine's effect on arrhythmias, Myers and Harris (1990) examined 35 patients with recent myocardial infarctions (within 5 to 10 days) in a double-blind crossover design. Patients received either 300 mg of caffeine plus an additional 150 mg of caffeine 4 hours later or a placebo. The researchers monitored the patients for 8 hours and then counted premature ventricular complexes (PVCs). They found no statistically significant difference in the number of PVCs. Goldberger remarked that PVCs are highly variable in general, which has always been problematic for studies on PVCs.

In another early study on arrhythmias, Chelsky et al. (1990) examined 222 patients, 86 percent with coronary artery disease and all habitual coffee users. All the patients were being evaluated for some sort of ventricular arrhythmia: nonsustained ventricular tachycardia, ventricular tachycardia, or ventricular fibrillation. The researchers attempted to induce very rapid rhythms in the patients' hearts both before and after caffeine consumption and found no difference in inducibility of ventricular arrhythmia on the basis of caffeine.

In what Goldberger described as a "curious" study of 600 patients who had experienced their first episode of atrial fibrillation, Mattioli et al. (2011) retrospectively examined caffeine intake in the days before the atrial fibrillation compared to usual intake. The researchers found that patients with moderately heavier caffeine use in the days prior to atrial fibrillation compared to usual intake had the lowest rate of successful spontaneous conversion to sinus rhythm. Patients with the lowest and highest intakes prior to atrial fibrillation had higher rates. The researchers called the response a U-shaped response.

In a 2011 review, Goldberger and Dan Pelchovitz (Pelchovitz and Goldberger, 2011) listed by size the studies they could find on the effect of caffeine on arrhythmia. Of those studies, three involved several thousand patients. Many more included far fewer numbers of patients. Goldberger highlighted one of the larger studies, the de Vreede-Swagemakers et al. (1999) study, which reported that, in a population with coronary artery disease (i.e., all the patients in the study had a clinical history of coronary artery disease), ingesting more than 10 cups of coffee per day was associated with an odds ratio of 55.7 for sudden cardiac death. This case-control study investigated 117 cases of sudden cardiac arrest and 144 controls, with controls matched by age and gender. A challenge for the investigators was to determine how many cups of coffee had been consumed by the patients who had died from sudden cardiac arrest. To answer that challenge, they asked the patients' relatives.

Thus, they also asked relatives of the controls how much coffee the controls had consumed. The researchers found dramatically fewer individuals in the control group who had consumed more than 10 cups of coffee per day, compared to individuals in the sudden cardiac arrest group. Interestingly, in Goldberger's opinion, what are typically considered risk factors, that is, hypercholesterolemia, diabetes mellitus, and smoking, were not identified as risk factors. The question for Goldberger is how to interpret such data given that they conflict with otherwise overwhelming data from other studies.

Since the Pelchovitz and Goldberger (2011) review, three additional observational studies involving thousands of patients have been published. Among all the observational studies conducted thus far, a total of about 315,000 patients have been evaluated. The average caffeine doses among these studies are consistent with information presented earlier during the workshop about amounts of caffeine intake (i.e., 2 cups of coffee daily: 148 mg/day for men, 285 mg/day for women; 5 cups daily: 274 mg/day for men and 232 mg/day for women), except a study conducted in Europe where average intake was greater (584 mg/day). Peak doses tend to be in 600 to 800 mg/day in the United States and greater than 1 g/day in Europe. According to Goldberger, the preponderance of these studies showed no increased risk of arrhythmias as a result of caffeine consumption.

The largest of these population studies, Klatsky et al. (2011), showed an inverse relationship between coffee intake and risk of hospitalization for arrhythmias, with an average follow-up of 17.6 years. That study was based on a Kaiser Permanente database of patients admitted to the hospital for arrhythmias. For "any arrhythmia," the odds ratio was 0.97 per cup per day, which represented a statistically significant decline as the number of cups of coffee per day increased. Odds ratios for several other diagnoses were either not significant or borderline significant. For premature beats, again the odds ratio, 0.87, represented a statistically significant decline in risk as coffee consumption increased. Whether the declines observed in Klatsky et al. (2011) are "real" is hard to know, in Goldberger's opinion. There are several caveats to population studies. Individuals who are sensitive to caffeine likely do not consume; there are ascertainment issues; exposure changes over time; source of caffeine varies and may matter, with other additives potentially having other effects; and most data do not include adolescents.

More broadly, there are studies that have examined other cardiovascular outcomes, some of which have shown negative outcomes in association with caffeine use and others positive outcomes. For example, Lopez-Garcia et al. (2006), a health professional's follow-up study, reported lower rates of coronary heart disease with caffeine consumption. But other studies have shown the opposite, according to Goldberger.

Conclusions About Caffeine and Arrhythmia Risk

Goldberger concluded by describing one final study, Graboys et al. (1989), of 50 individuals, all with significant arrhythmias and structural heart disease. The individuals were administered caffeine on one day and no caffeine on a successive day. The researchers found that caffeine and catecholamine levels increased with caffeine consumption, as expected, but they observed no change in PVCs with caffeine consumption. The researchers concluded, "Although patients with cardiac disease are frequently warned about the potential harmful effects of caffeine, this clinical advice is based primarily on anecdote and folklore" (p. 639). That was 25 years ago. In Goldberger's opinion, some data today suggest that caffeine effects are present, but the prevailing evidence shows no increase in arrhythmia. Moreover, what effects do exist are dose dependent and different in habitual versus nonhabitual users. Researchers have demonstrated mild changes in hemodynamic parameters (heart rate and blood pressure), a slight increase in sympathetic activity, and small changes in cardiac electrophysiologic properties.

CAFFEINE AND POTENTIAL RISK OF HYPERTENSION

Presented by Ahmed El-Sohemy, Ph.D.,
University of Toronto

In Ahmed El-Sohemy's opinion, the marketing of energy drinks to children and adolescents is a major issue. Isolated case reports of premature death following consumption of an energy drink usually occur in the context of some kind of physical exertion or activity and primarily among youth and adolescents. Despite denials by some manufacturers, El-Sohemy opined, it is difficult to argue that such drinks are not intended to appeal to youth. For example, recently at a high school in Winnipeg, Canada, an energy drink company was distributing certificates containing advertising messages to graduating students. Many of those students were under the age of 18.

El-Sohemy showed some slides courtesy of Jim Shepherd, whose son died a few years ago at a paintball event. Although the finding was not conclusive, there was reason to believe that consumption of an energy drink at that event, which was the first time Shepherd's son had consumed one, may have triggered the fatal cardiac event. The slides contained images of some of the products and ways that El-Sohemy believes they are being marketed to youth. For example, a product that El-Sohemy said was taken off the shelves had a label at the top of the can that read, "The Legal Alternative." That sort of marketing appeals to risk-taking behavior, in El-Sohemy's opinion. Other types of caffeinated products on the shelves are of concern, too, El-Sohemy said. These products include brownies, gummy bears, potato chips, and gum. The *Lancet* published a case report several years ago describing the hospitalization of a 13-year-old boy with tachycardia and elevated blood pressure (Natale et al., 2009). The boy had consumed 2 packs of gum containing 160 mg of caffeine. There was good evidence, according to El-Sohemy, that consumption of the gum was responsible for the cardiovascular event that required hospitalization.

Globally, coffee is "still king" with respect to caffeine exposure, El-Sohemy said. Coffee is the second most widely traded commodity, after oil. Among adults in many parts of the world, coffee is still the biggest source of caffeine. Of course, El-Sohemy observed, a cup of coffee is no longer "just a cup of coffee." For example, Tim Hortons (a restaurant chain in Canada and the United States) recently added a new extra-large-sized coffee, a 24-ounce cup containing several hundred milligrams of caffeine. El-Sohemy pointed this out because many energy drink manufacturers have argued that if energy drinks are going to be regulated, then coffee should be regulated too because many cans of energy drinks have an equivalent amount of caffeine as a cup of coffee. In fact, they argue that some cups of coffee have more caffeine than what is found in energy drinks. However, it is important to note, El-Sohemy said, that a distinction exists between caffeine from energy drinks and caffeine from coffee. Caffeine is caffeine from a chemical structure perspective, but there is a big difference in terms of peak concentrations of caffeine between slowly sipping a hot beverage versus chugging a cold beverage.

Is Coffee Associated with Cardiovascular Disease?

Dozens of studies have examined the association between coffee and cardiovascular disease. Not surprisingly, in El-Sohemy's opinion, some have shown an increased risk of cardiovascular disease with caffeine exposure, others have shown no effect, and yet others have shown a decreased effect with moderate consumption. Some studies have shown a U-shaped or J-shaped association, with moderate consumption associated with the lowest risk. There are many possible reasons for these inconsistencies. One is the genetic background of the population being studied. El-Sohemy and his research team wanted to explore the possibility that individuals with certain genotypes are more vulnerable and at greater risk while individuals with certain other genotypes experience no effect or might actually benefit from moderate consumption.

El-Sohemy explained that he and his team were interested specifically in caffeine. After all, he said, coffee is a complex beverage with many kinds of bioactive substances. Some, such as the polyphenols, with their antioxidant properties, are believed to have beneficial effects, whereas others, such as the diterpenoids, which are known to raise low-density lipoprotein cholesterol, could have adverse effects.

Caffeine is broken down almost exclusively by the drug-metabolizing liver enzyme CYP1A2 and converted into a more water-soluble compound, paraxanthine, which itself is rapidly broken down into other water-soluble compounds. CYP1A2 catalyzes the rate-limiting detoxification of caffeine, with the gene that codes for CYP1A2 having a common polymorphism (–163 A/C) with a profound effect on enzyme activity. Carriers of the C allele are slow metabolizers. Individuals homozygous for the A allele have a fourfold higher rate of caffeine metabolism. El-Sohemy's team reasoned that if caffeine is a component in coffee that could increase the risk of heart attack, then slow metabolizers should be at higher risk than fast metabolizers because caffeine lingers longer in slow metabolizers' systems.

As described in Cornelis et al. (2006), El-Sohemy and colleagues examined genetic variation in CYP1A2 and coffee intake in more than two thousand cases of a first acute myocardial infarction and an equal number of controls matched for age, sex, and area of residence. They used a food frequency questionnaire to assess coffee consumption and other sources of caffeine. They found that 90 percent of caffeine intake came from coffee. They genotyped participants from fasting blood samples. Without taking genetics into account, but taking into account potential confounding factors such as smoking, physical activity, and saturated fat intake, the researchers found that consuming four or more cups of coffee a day was associated with about a 36 percent increased risk of a myocardial infarction and a statistically significant odds ratio of 1.36.

El-Sohemy explained that, if they had stopped their research with that finding, they would have concluded that drinking four or more cups of coffee per day is associated with an increased risk of a heart attack. But the real question they wanted to address was related to caffeine intake and its association with myocardial infarction. Again, if caffeine increases the risk, then one would expect slow metabolizers to be at a higher risk. Indeed, that is what they found when they stratified the study population by CYP1A2 genotype (see Figure 5-1). Among slow metabolizers, two to three cups of coffee per day was associated with a significantly increased risk. Among the fast metabolizers, there was no increased risk. If anything, the data show signs of a U-shaped association, according to El-Sohemy.

At the time those data were collected, researchers believed that that caffeine more likely acted as a trigger of cardiovascular disease among younger individuals in particular. As expected, Cornelis et al. (2006) observed a shift in odds ratios for subjects younger than 50 years of age (see Figure 5-1), with slow metabolizers showing a more pronounced risk of heart attack, almost a fourfold increased risk, and with a significant protective effect of moderate consumption among fast metabolizers. El-Sohemy suspects that, at moderate levels of consumption, fast metabolizers are able to efficiently eliminate the caffeine, which would otherwise be masking some of the beneficial effects of the polyphenols and other bioactive substances. But once these individuals reach four or more cups a day, even though they are fast metabolizers, their CYP1A2 enzyme begins to become saturated so that the adverse effects of caffeine begin to counter the beneficial effects of the polyphenols and other compounds.

El-Sohemy reiterated that the only difference between slow and fast metabolizers who drink four or more cups a day of coffee in Cornelis et al. (2006) is a single nucleotide polymorphism that affects the rate at which caffeine is eliminated from the body. Because caffeine is the only major substance in coffee that is known to be detoxified by CYP1A2, the findings strongly implicate caffeine as a trigger for the increased risk of heart attack.

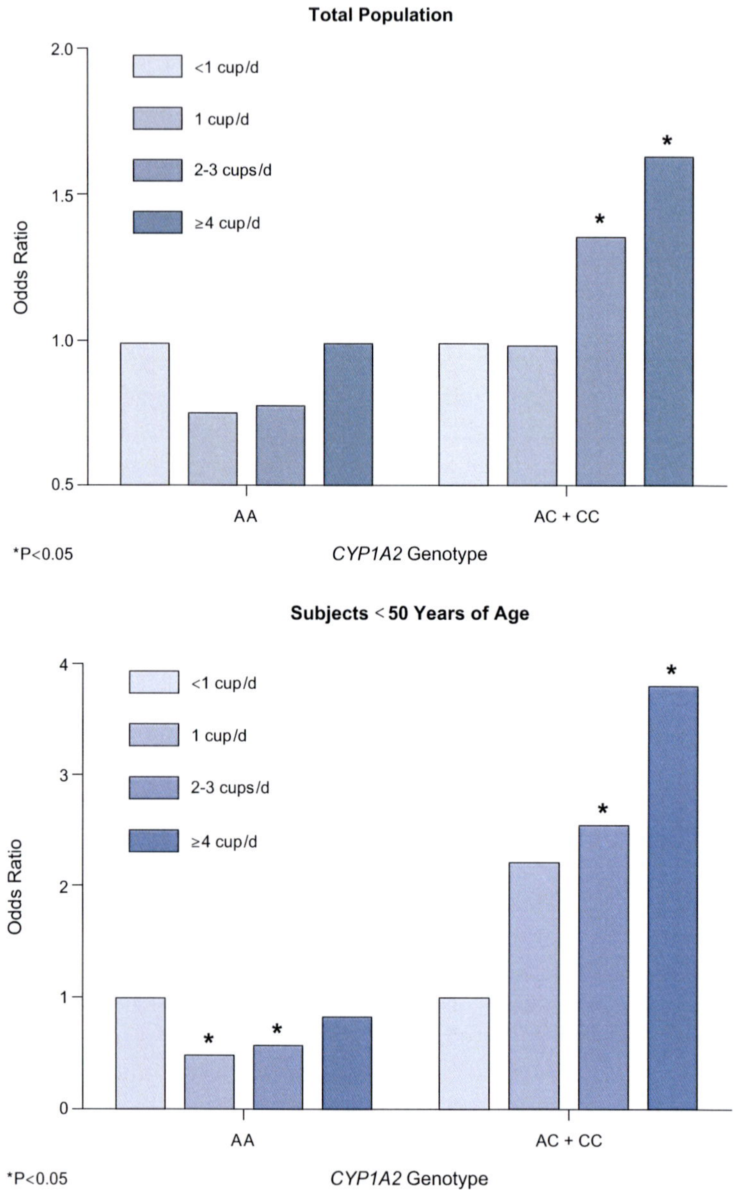

FIGURE 5-1 Odds ratios of risk of myocardial infarction with coffee intake.
NOTES: AA = fast caffeine metabolizer, AC + CC = slow caffeine metabolizer. Top panel: all study participants; bottom panel: study participants less than 50 years of age.
SOURCE: Cornelis et al., 2006.

As El-Sohemy noted, that study attracted a lot of media attention, with headlines reading, "Why two cups of coffee can damage your heart" and "Gene that could make your next coffee your last." But it wasn't until a few years later that another research group built on the findings by examining whether CYP1A2 might also explain some of the inconsistencies in studies linking coffee to risk of hypertension (Palatini et al., 2009). They essentially achieved the same results, with an increased risk of hypertension as coffee consumption increases among slow metabolizers but with a decreased risk of hypertension among fast metabolizers. Again, if genetics were not taken into account, one would conclude that coffee has no effect on hypertension. The study was prospective. The researchers examined prehypertensive individuals, genotyped them, and followed them. They also investigated the relationship between CYP1A2 genotype and catecholamines and, again, found that epinephrine concentrations increased with increased coffee consumption only among the slow metabolizers.

In another example of the importance of genetic variation in understanding the cardiovascular risks associated with caffeine consumption, a research group in Finland reported that genetic variation in the catechol-O-methyltransferase (COMT) gene, which is involved in the metabolism of catecholamines such as epinephrine, is associated with varying risk of acute coronary events (Happonen et al., 2006). Specifically, they found that individuals with the genotype associated with high COMT activity showed no increased risk with increased coffee consumption but that individuals with the genotype associated with low COMT activity did show an increased risk with increased coffee consumption. More recently, Brathwaite et al. (2011) reported that COMT could also explain why some people experience increased heart rate following caffeine consumption.

Personalized Dietary Advice Versus Public Health Recommendations

El-Sohemy concluded by emphasizing the importance of individual variation and the challenge of reconciling public health advice with personalized dietary advice. A "one-size-fits-all" approach clearly does not apply when it comes to caffeine consumption. There are probably many other genetic variants, in addition to those described here, that explain other types of responses. In El-Sohemy's opinion, it is highly unlikely that the several cases of premature death following the consumption of energy drinks are caused by CYP1A2 variation, which is very common in the population, or COMT variation, which is also fairly common. But it is likely that the cases are caused by some other genetic variant. He said, "But what we don't know is how common that other genetic variant is because it has not yet been identified." In terms of regulation, he stressed the importance of taking into account these vulnerable (genetic) subgroups and ensuring that they are protected.

PANELIST DISCUSSION WITH THE AUDIENCE

Following El-Sohemy's presentation, workshop participants were invited to ask questions of the three panelists. Most of the discussion revolved around the future research needs on the cardiovascular effects of caffeine exposure, including in vulnerable populations, and differences between caffeine in energy drinks versus coffee.

Future Research Needs

Some workshop participants expressed disagreement regarding the urgency of concern with consumption of energy drinks, with one audience member remarking that he has not seen "in the real clinical world" the adverse effects being studied in the lab. He suggested that if a problem with energy drink consumption did exist, more people would be admitted for arrhythmias, heart attacks, and so forth. In response, Higgins explained that, as some workshop presenters emphasized, not all individuals are equal. It may be that the cardiologists who treat adults are not seeing the same problems that the cardiologists who treat children are seeing. Some people may be vulnerable by age, others by exposure to caffeine, and still others because of a genetic predisposition. Also, the substrates are different. In his opinion, coffee, with its many antioxidants and other components, is not the same as pure caffeine. Nor are either coffee or pure caffeine equal to caffeine-containing energy drinks. He said that "obviously more research is needed" with respect to why some individuals have greater reactions than others.

Goldberger added that, although there are no large differences in arrhythmia on a population level, nonetheless he occasionally comes across patients with arrhythmias who report sensitivity to caffeine. In addition to genetic factors, other factors may to help identify the small subset of individuals who are more susceptible to arrhythmias on exposure to caffeine.

Goldberger was asked whether any of the studies he described involved individuals under the age of 18 and whether any of the studies differentiated between caffeine versus coffee versus energy drinks versus other energy products. Goldberger replied that the preponderance of population studies have examined coffee intake, with not much additional information available. Most have not addressed vulnerable populations.

Implications of a Study with an "N" of One

One audience member expressed concern that a sample size of 1 (i.e., Higgins's SHADE-ONE study) does not reflect "true variation" and stressed the importance of replication before drawing generalizations. He wondered what the ECF response would be in a large population and how ECF would vary in response to different doses. Higgins cited Worthley et al. (2010), a study with an N of 50, which presented clear evidence of endothelial dysfunction as measured by reactive hyperemia and platelet aggregation. He remarked that there are other larger (i.e., larger than N = 1) studies as well and that the pilot study he mentioned with an N of one (Higgins, 2013) is currently being followed up with a larger study with an N of about 50.

Different Studies Have Different End Points

Yet another audience member observed that Higgins's research "flies in the face of decades of research showing that caffeine actually increases performance." Higgins explained that his research on ECF does not relate to performance. He did not disagree with the audience member's claim about other studies on performance, but he has been looking only at arterial function.

Differences Between Caffeine in Energy Drinks Versus Coffee

One audience member disputed El-Sohemy's claim that peak concentrations from chugging a cold drink are different from those from slowly sipping a hot beverage. According to the audience member, the dose response is the same for similar doses regardless of whether the dose is being consumed slowly or quickly. El-Sohemy replied that the actual dose, the actual amount of caffeine being consumed, is not the only issue. In terms of peak plasma concentrations, which can have important physiological effects, chugging a cold beverage leads to a higher peak plasma concentration and could have a profound effect even if the dose is smaller than the dose in a hot beverage sipped slowly.

REFERENCES

Bellet, S., E. Horstmann, L. R. Roman, N. T. DeGuzman, and J. B. Kostis. 1972. Effect of caffeine on the ventricular fibrillation threshold in normal dogs and dogs with acute myocardial infarction. *American Heart Journal* 84:215–227.

Brathwaite, J. M., L. A. Da Costa, and A. El-Sohemy. 2011. Catechol-o-methyltransferase genotype is associated with self-reported increased heart rate following caffeine consumption. *Journal of Caffeine Research* 1:123–130.

Chelsky, L. B., J. E. Cutler, K. Griffith, J. Kron, J. H. McClelland, and J. H. McAnulty. 1990. Caffeine and ventricular arrhythmias: An electrophysiologic approach. *Journal of the American Medical Association* 264:2236–2240.

Cornelis, M. C., A. El-Sohemy, E. K. Kabagambe, and H. Campos. 2006. Coffee, CYP1A2 genotype, and risk of myocardial infarction. *Journal of the American Medical Association* 295:1135–1141.

Corti, R., C. Binggeli, I. Sudano, L. Spieker, E. Hänseler, F. Ruschitzka, W. F. Chaplin, T. F. Lüschers, and G. Noll. 2002. Coffee acutely increases sympathetic nerve activity and blood pressure independently of caffeine content: Role of habitual versus nonhabitual drinking. *Circulation* 106:2935–2940.

De Vreede-Swagemakers, J. J., A. P. Gorgels, M. P. Weijenberg, W. I. Dubois-Arbouw, B. Golombeck, J. W. van Ree, A. Knottnerus, and H. J. Wellens. 1999. Risk indicators for out-of-hospital cardiac arrest in patients with coronary artery disease. *Journal of Clinical Epidemiology* 52:601–607.

Echeverri, D., F. R. Montes, M. Cabrera, A. Galán, and A. Prieto. 2010. Caffeine's vascular mechanisms of action. *International Journal of Vascular Medicine* article ID: 834060. doi: 10.1155/2010/834060. PMCID: PMC3003984.

Graboys, T. B., C. M. Blatt, and B. Lown. 1989. The effect of caffeine on ventricular ectopic activity in patients with malignant ventricular arrhythmia. *Archives of Internal Medicine* 149:637–639.

Happonen, P., S. Voutilainen, T. P. Tuomainen, and J. T. Salonen. 2006. Catechol-o-methyltransferase gene polymorphism modifies the effect of coffee intake on incidence of acute coronary events. *PLoS ONE* (1):e117. doi: 10 1371/journqlpone 0000117.

Higgins, J. P. 2013. Endothelial function acutely worse after drinking energy beverage. *International Journal of Cardiology*. http://www.sciencedirect.com/science/article/pii/S0167527313011728.

Higgins, J. P., and K. M. Babu. 2013. Caffeine reduces myocardial blood flow during exercise. *American Journal of Medicine* 126(8):730.e731–730.e738.

Hughes, J. R., G. Amori, and D. K. Hatsukami. 1988. A survey of physician advice about caffeine. *Journal of Substance Abuse* 1:67–70.

Jackman, M., P. Wendling, D. Friars, and T. E. Graham. 1996. Metabolic catecholamine, and endurance responses to caffeine during intense exercise. *Journal of Applied Physiology* 81:1658–1663.

Klatsky, A. L., A. S. Hasan, M. A. Armstrong, N. Udaltsova, and C. Morton. 2011. Coffee, caffeine, and risk of hospitalization for arrhythmias. *Permanente Journal* 15:19–25.

Lee, R., K. M. Channon, and C. Antoniades. 2012. Therapeutic strategies targeting endothelial function in humans: Clinical implications. *Current Vascular Pharmacology* 10:77–93

Lopez-Garcia, E., R. M. van Dam, W. C. Willett, E. B. Rimm, J. E. Manson, M. J. Stampfer, K. M. Rexrode, and F. B. Hu. 2006. Coffee consumption and coronary heart disease in men and women: A prospective cohort study. *Circulation* 113:2045–2053.

Mattioli, A. V., A. Farinetti, C. Miloro, P. Pedrazzi, and G. Mattioli. 2011. Influence of coffee and caffeine consumption on atrial fibrillation in hypertensive patients. *Nutrition, Metabolism, and Cardiovascular Diseases* 21:412–417.

Myers, M. G., and L. Harris. 1990. High dose caffeine and ventricular arrhythmias. *Canadian Journal of Cardiology* 6:95–98.

Natale, F., C. Cirillos, G. M. Di Marco, L. S. di Vetta, L. Aronne, A. Siciliano, R. Mocerino, M. A. Tedesco, P. Golino, and R. Calabrò. 2009. When chewing gum is more than just a bad habit. *Lancet* 373:1918.

Palatini, P., G. Ceolotto, F. Ragazzo, F. Dorigatti, F. Saladini, I. Papparella, L. Mos, G. Zanata, and M. Santonastaso. 2009. CYP1A2 genotype modifies the association between coffee intake and the risk of hypertension. *Journal of Hypertension* 27:1594–1601.

Pelchovitz, D. J., and J. J. Goldberger. 2011. Caffeine and cardiac arrhythmias: A review of the evidence. *American Journal of Medicine* 124:284–289.

Rashid, A., M. Hines, B. J. Scherlag, W. S. Yamanashi, and W. Lovallo. 2006. The effects of caffeine on the inducibility of atrial fibrillation. *Journal of Electrocardiology* 39:421–425.

Sumpio, B. E., J. T. Riley, and A. Dardik. 2002. Cells in focus: Endothelial cell. *International Journal of Biochemistry and Cell Biology* 34:1508–1512.

Widlansky, M. E., N. Gokce, J. F. Keaney, Jr., and J. A. Vita. 2003. The clinical implications of endothelial dysfunction. *Journal of the American College of Cardiology* 42:1149–1160.

Worthley, M. I., A. Prabhus, P. De Sciscio, C. Schultz, P. Sanders, and S. R. Willoughby. 2010. Detrimental effects of energy drink consumption on platelet and endothelial function. *American Journal of Medicine* 123:184–187.

6

Caffeine Effects on the Central Nervous System and Behavioral Effects Associated with Caffeine Consumption

In addition to its potential impact on cardiac health, public health experts are concerned about the effect of high levels of caffeine exposure on the central nervous system and behavior. In the Day 1, Session 4, panel, moderated by Thomas J. Gould, Ph.D., Department of Psychology, Temple University, Philadelphia, Pennsylvania, panelists explored scientific evidence on the effects of caffeine exposure on the central nervous system. In the Day 1, Session 5, panel, moderated by Richard H. Adamson, Ph.D., TPN Associates, panelists considered the behavioral effects of caffeine consumption. This chapter summarizes the panelists' presentations in both sessions and the discussions that followed. Because of the similarity in topics, also included in this chapter is a summary of Andrew Smith's presentation from Day 2, Session 2. Box 6-1 describes the key points made by each speaker.

MECHANISMS OF THE CENTRAL NERVOUS SYSTEM EFFECTS OF CAFFEINE

Presented by Sergi Ferré, Ph.D., M.D., National Institute on Drug Abuse

Caffeine is a psychostimulant with the same central effects as the classical nervous system psychostimulants cocaine and amphetamine, according to Sergi Ferré. That is, it increases motor activity and has both arousal and reinforcing effects, although its reinforcing effects are not as strong as those of the classical psychostimulants. But its mechanism of action is different. Ferré provided an overview of research conducted since the early 1990s on the mechanism of action of caffeine on the central nervous system.

BOX 6-1

Key Points Made by Individual Speakers

- Sergi Ferré described caffeine as a psychostimulant with the same central nervous system effects as classical psychostimulants such as cocaine and amphetamine. That is, it increases motor activity, induces arousal, and creates reinforcing effects. Its mechanism of action is different, however. Ferré explained how caffeine exerts its psychostimulant effects by blocking adenosine receptors.
- Jennifer Temple noted that most studies on the psychopharmacological and other physiological effects of caffeine have been conducted on adults. Temple described her research group's work on behavioral and cardiac effects in children and adolescents. Many of her findings are consistent with what has been found in adults, except for a lack of difference in response between low versus high caffeine users. Of note, boys appear to be more responsive to caffeine than girls are.
- Roland Griffiths brought up the point that scientists have conducted numerous studies on the behavioral effects of caffeine exposure, including its reinforcing effects (the self-administration of caffeine), tolerance (reduced responsiveness due to drug exposure), physical dependence (withdrawal), and addiction ("DSM [*Diagnostic and Statistical Manual*] dependence syndrome").
- Both Griffiths and Charles O'Brien explained how the growing evidence base for caffeine withdrawal led to it being recognized as a diagnosis in the fifth edition of the DSM (DSM-5). Griffiths expressed concern that withdrawal-sensitive youth who experience delays or disruptions in their habitual pattern of intake will likely experience adverse emotional, cognitive, and behavioral consequences.
- Caffeine addiction, on the other hand, is not as well studied and thus not recognized as a diagnosis in DSM-5. But caffeine addiction is recommended as a diagnosis for further study. O'Brien emphasized the individual variation in the behavioral effects of caffeine exposure and suggested that caffeine addiction may have a genetic basis.
- Amelia Arria said the consumption of caffeinated energy drinks was first associated with risk-taking behavior in 1996. Arria discussed evidence that has accumulated since then and the rising concerns among public health professionals that the possible contribution of caffeinated energy-drink consumption to risk-taking behavior may have health and safety consequences for adolescents and young adults.

- Andrew Smith said that beginning in the 1990s, scientists have demonstrated beneficial effects of caffeine exposure alongside their negative effects. Indeed, in Smith's opinion, the levels of caffeine consumed by most people have largely beneficial effects on alertness, attention, and other behaviors. Smith cautioned, however, that excessive consumption can cause problems in children and other sensitive individuals.

Research in the Early 1990s

Ferré said that it is well known that the mechanism underlying the motor and reinforcing effects of cocaine and amphetamine are caused by the drugs' stimulation of central dopaminergic transmission, particularly in the striatum. The striatum, the input structure of the basal ganglia, is an area of the brain involved in the elicitation and learning of reward-related behaviors, and it contains the highest concentration of dopamine and dopamine receptors. Cocaine and amphetamine are able to produce psychostimulant effects by binding to what is known as a dopamine transporter and either blocking (e.g., cocaine) or reversing (e.g., amphetamine) its effects. In both cases, the end result is a significant increase of dopamine in the extracellular space, which in turn activates the postsynaptic dopamine D1 and D2 receptors.

In contrast to cocaine and amphetamine, in the early 1990s scientists already knew that the main mechanism underlying caffeine psychostimulation was adenosine receptor antagonism. It was known then that caffeine at brain concentrations obtained after drinking coffee was enough to block the effects of the A1 and A2A receptors, with A2B being involved only in pathological situations and A3 having little affinity for caffeine. (There are four adenosine receptors: A1, A2A, A2B, and A3.) The question then was, How does adenosine modulate the dopaminergic system?

Also in the 1990s, scientists were aware that caffeine does not produce a clear or strong presynaptic dopamine-releasing effect. That is, it does not really increase dopamine in the extracellular space in the brain. Knowing that, Ferré and collaborators investigated the possibility of a postsynaptic interaction between adenosine and dopamine receptor signaling (Ferré et al., 1991a). They used the reserpinized mouse model to test their hypothesis. (Reserpine depletes dopamine and other catecholamines in the brain, resulting in an animal becoming immobile, or cataleptic. The only way to counteract the catatelptic effect is to administer a dopamine receptor agonist, that is, something that stimulates the postsynaptic dopaminergic receptors.) They used bromocriptine (a D2 agonist) to produce locomotor activity in reserpinized mice. They found that the locomotor effect of bromocriptine was counteracted by the adenosine receptor agonists NECA (an A1/A2A agonist) and L-PIA (an A1 agonist) with a potency that suggested predominant involvement of A2A receptors.

Ferré and collaborators (1991a) also found that caffeine (an A1/A2A agonist) and caffeine metabolites theophylline (an A1/A2A agonist) and paraxanthine, but not theobromine, had the opposite effect; that is, they potentiated locomotor activity of bromocriptine. That finding suggested the existence of an antagonistic interaction between the postsynaptic adenosine A2A and dopamine D2 receptors, through which A2A receptor agonists would behave as D2 receptor antagonists, and A2A receptor antagonists would behave as dopamine as D2 receptor agonists. Indeed, in a separate study, Ferré et al. (1991b) demonstrated for the first time that central administration of an A2A receptor agonist would produce catalepsy, as a dopamine D2 receptor antagonist would do. Later, when selective adenosine A2A receptor antagonists became available, others demonstrated the opposite effect: that A2A receptor antagonists elicit motor activation (Karcz-Kubicha et al., 2003).

The findings reported in Ferré et al. (1991a,b) strongly suggested that caffeine produces motor activation by blocking adenosine A2A receptor–mediated inhibition of dopamine D2 receptor activation. Later, through radioligand-binding experimentation, Ferré and his team found evidence for a more direct interaction between the two receptors (Ferré et al., 1991c), with the dopamine D2 receptor antagonist being displaced by dopamine in a dose-dependent manner and with the ability of dopamine to displace the antagonist being modified by the addition of an adenosine A2A receptor agonist (CGS21680). That is, the agonist CGS21680 decreased the affinity of dopamine D2 receptors for dopamine. That experiment also demonstrated that the A2A and D2 receptors should be localized in the same neuron. But which neuron was it?

Subsequent study pointed to the efferent striatal gamma-aminobutyric acid (GABA)-ergic medium spiny neuron, also known as MSN. MSNs are efferent neurons that constitute more than 95 percent of the striatal neuronal population. They receive two main inputs: glutamatergic inputs from the cortical-limbic-thalamic area and mesencephalic dopaminergic inputs from the substantia nigra and ventral tegmental area.

There are two subtypes of MSNs, each of which gives rise to a separate efferent pathway connecting the striatum with the output structures of the basal ganglia (i.e., the medial segment of the globus pallidus and the substantia nigra pars reticulate). One of the pathways is direct, the other indirect. Using freely moving rats, Ferré et al. (1993) inserted one probe into the striatum, where cell bodies of the indirect MSN are localized, and another probe into the ipsilateral global pallidus, where the nerve terminals of the indirect MSN are localized and where GABA is released. They found that perfusion of a D2 receptor agonist, pergolide, through the striatal probe resulted in a significant reduction of extracellular levels of GABA in the ipsilateral globus pallidus. The effect was significantly counteracted by the striatal coperfusion of an A2A receptor agonist, CGS21680, and significantly potentiated by the xanthine theophylline.

Two New Concepts

Ferré described what he said were two new concepts being used in pharmacology to help explain the central mechanism of action of caffeine and many other compounds: receptor heteromer and local module. The receptor concept was introduced in 1878; since then, receptors have been considered as single functional units. But that view is changing. A receptor heteromer is defined as a macromolecular complex composed of at least two functional receptor units with biochemical properties that are demonstrably different from those of its individual components (Ferré et al., 2009).

The second concept, local module, relates to the MSN and the convergence of MSN's two main inputs (i.e., the cortical-limbic-thalamic glutamatergic terminal making synaptic contact with the head of the dendritic spine and the mesencephalic dopaminergic terminal making synaptic contact with the neck of the dendritic spine). Together, these various elements—the dendritic spine, the glutamatergic terminal, dopaminergic terminal, and glial processes that wrap around the glutamatergic synapse—constitute a functional unit known as the striatal spine module, a type of local module. A local module is defined as the minimal portion of one or more neurons and/or one or more glial cells that operates as an independent integrative unit (Ferré et al., 2007).

As described by Ferré, the concept of a local module provides a framework for understanding the functional roles of extrasynaptic transmission. Dopamine is released not only intrasynaptically, but also extrasynaptically, which allows activation of extrasynaptic receptors localized at dopamine and glutamate synapses and modulation of glutamatergic neurotransmission. The same is true of glutamate. It is not only released intrasynaptically but also spills over and stimulates extrasynaptic glutamate receptors localized at glutamate and dopaminergic synapses and modulates dopaminergic neurotransmission. Extrasynaptic transmission and extrasynaptic localization of receptors, in turn, provide a framework for understanding the existence and possible functional role of receptor heteromers.

According to Ferré, much work has been done using artificial systems and resonance energy transfer techniques (BRET and FRET), as well as mass spectrometry analysis of peptide-peptide interactions, to demonstrate the formation of A2A-D2 receptor heteromers (Canals et al., 2003; Woods and Ferré, 2005; Navarro et al., 2010). Ferré and his colleagues have used patch-clamp experiments (i.e., with transgenic mice that express green fluorescent protein and show fluorescence in the D2 receptor–containing neuron) to gain an understanding of these interactions at the cellular level. Specifically, they have shown that the N-methyl-D-aspartate (NMDA) receptor induces strong activation, an effect that is completely inhibited by the D2 receptor agonist *N*-1-naphthylphthalamic acid (NPA) and that the A2A receptor agonist CGS21680, which by itself does not produce any effect, completely counteracts the D2 receptor–mediated inhibition (Azdad et al., 2009). Furthermore, Azdad et al. (2009) found that infusing a peptide corresponding to an A2A receptor epitope involved in A2A-D2 receptor heteromerization interrupts the antagonistic interaction between the A2A and D2 receptors.

Other Mechanisms of Caffeine Psychostimulant Effects

In Ferré's opinion, scientists have reached a high level of understanding of at least one mechanism of action of caffeine: the A2A-D2 antagonistic interaction mediated by the A2A-D2 receptor heteromer localized in the indirect MSN. The mechanism explains not only the motor-depressant effects of A2A receptor agonists but also the motor-activating effects of caffeine and other A2A receptor antagonists (Orrú et al., 2011). On the basis of this knowledge, researchers have been testing the efficacy of A2A receptor antagonists in the treatment of Parkinson's disease.

Not all caffeine effects are mediated by A2A, according to Ferré. Some motor effects are mediated by the A1 receptor (Karcz-Kubicha et al., 2003). Ferré did not elaborate, but he did remark that the same methods were used to identify an antagonistic A1-D1 receptor interaction in the direct MSN that also mediates the postsynaptic effects of caffeine (Ferré et al., 1996).

In addition to postsynaptic mechanisms, presynaptic mechanism could also be involved in caffeine's locomotor-activating effects. Although no evidence indicates that caffeine releases dopamine like cocaine and amphetamine do, Solinas et al. (2002) showed that it does release dopamine in the very ventral part of the striatum, in an area called the shell of the nucleus accumbens, by acting on adenosine A1 receptors localized in glutamatergic and dopamatergic terminals.

A final mechanism for the motor and probably reinforcing effects of caffeine was recently described in the literature (Ferré et al., 2013; Orrú et al., 2013). It involves paraxanthine, the main metabolite of caffeine in humans, which has a very strong psychostimulant effect in rats and is correlated with a significant dopamine release in striatal areas of the brain where caffeine is ineffective. Ferré and his team learned that paraxanthine has a unique pharmacological profile. In addition to being an A1 and A2A receptor antagonist, it is also a selective inhibitor of cGMP-preferring phosphodiesterase (PDE) and thus plays a role in potentiating nitrous oxide transmission.

Most of the mechanisms that Ferré discussed were relevant to the motor and reinforcing effects of caffeine. Arousal is another central effect of caffeine that, according to Ferré, seems to be related to multiple interconnected ascending arousal systems moderated by adenosine A1 receptors (Ferré, 2010).

Conclusions About the Neurological Effects of Caffeine

Ferré concluded with four main summary points:

1. Two new concepts, "receptor heteromer" and "local module," facilitate the understanding of the functional role of interactions between neurotransmitters and receptor heteromers in the central nervous system and of the mechanisms of caffeine and other central-acting drugs.

2. The motor and rewarding effects of caffeine depend on its ability to release the pre- and post-synaptic brakes that adenosine imposes on dopaminergic neurotransmission by acting on different adenosine A2A and A1 receptor heteromers localized in different elements of the striatal spine module.
3. The arousal effects of caffeine depend on its ability to release the A1 receptor-mediated inhibitory modulation of the highly interconnected multiple ascending arousal systems.
4. Paraxanthine, the main metabolite of caffeine in humans, displays a strong psychostimulant profile that depends on its selective ability to potentiate nitric oxide neurotransmission.

DEVELOPMENTAL AND PSYCHOPHARMACOLOGICAL EFFECTS OF CAFFEINE

Presented by Jennifer Temple, Ph.D., University of Buffalo

Caffeine has many physiological effects, both acute (e.g., cardiovascular, ergogenic) and chronic (e.g., tolerance and withdrawal) (Bender et al., 1997; Fredholm et al., 1999; Wesensten et al., 2002; Waring et al., 2003; Davis and Green, 2009; Juliano et al., 2012; Rogers et al., 2013). Caffeine also has many well-described psychopharmacological effects, including increased energy (Griffiths et al., 1990), increased alertness (Haskell et al., 2008), improved mood (Garrett and Griffiths, 1998), and enhanced cognitive performance (Smit and Rogers, 2000). According to Jennifer Temple, most studies on the effects of caffeine have been conducted in adults. Temple presented data from her research on the effects of caffeine in children and adolescents.

First, however, she remarked on variation in caffeine use. Not only does the dosage of caffeine vary widely across sources, with several coffees and energy drinks exceeding the FDA limit for caffeine in cola, but caffeine use patterns vary across the lifespan. Average daily caffeine consumption increases and peaks in the 35- to 54-year-old age group and then tapers off (Frary et al., 2005). More important for Temple's research, dietary sources of caffeine also vary across the lifespan. According to data collected between 1994 and 1998 and reported in Frary et al. (2005), the primary source of caffeine for children under the age of 18 is soda, with very little coffee consumption, with a big shift occurring after the age of 18, when coffee becomes the primary source of caffeine. That finding does not take into account energy drinks; Temple suspected that the data would show a slightly different pattern if energy drinks were included.

Three Vulnerable Populations

From the perspective of caffeine use, Temple identified three vulnerable populations: (1) pregnant women, with some evidence that excessive caffeine may increase the risk of miscarriage but with little known about the effects of caffeine use during pregnancy on offspring later in life; (2) children, because of their exposure to high doses in terms of milligrams of caffeine per kilogram of body weight and because caffeine may be a gateway to other substances; and (3) adolescents, because of escalating use during adolescence and the combining of energy drinks and alcohol.

Focusing just on children and adolescents, Temple identified three main differences between those two populations and adults that explain why she considers children and adolescents to be vulnerable populations. First, sources of caffeine are different, again with children and adolescents drinking more soda and adults drinking more coffee. Although the caffeine content of coffee can vary on the basis of how it is brewed and where it is purchased, nonetheless caffeine is a natural component of coffee. Soda and energy drinks do not naturally contain caffeine. Rather, those beverages are vehicles for caffeine. A second difference is that the lifetime experience with caffeine is very different in children than in adults. Most adults consume caffeine and have had a history of caffeine use, which affords them some tolerance to the effects of caffeine. In contrast, children, especially young children, are fairly naïve with respect to caffeine use. They tend to consume caffeine at relatively low doses and with less frequency or less regularity than adults do, which may make them particularly vulnerable to the effects of a large amount of caffeine consumed at once. A third difference is that children's and adolescents' brains are still developing, especially in the frontal lobe, with little known about the impact of high levels of caffeine on the brain during this critical period of brain development.

Evidence on the Effects of Caffeine in Children and Adolescents

When Temple and her colleagues first starting studying the effects of caffeine in children and adolescents, about 7 years ago, so little research had been conducted that she felt as though they were starting from scratch. Her research has focused on four main areas: reinforcing properties of caffeine, cardiovascular responses to caffeine, subjective effects of caffeine, and cognitive effects of caffeine. She discussed each in turn.

Reinforcing Properties of Caffeine

Curious about why manufacturers would add caffeine to soda, Temple and her team first conducted studies on the reinforcing properties of caffeine. The claim from beverage manufacturers is that caffeine is added to enhance flavor. But caffeine has an extremely bitter flavor, and at the levels of caffeine added to sodas, studies have shown that few people can taste the difference between caffeinated and noncaffeinated soda. Temple and her colleagues approached this work with the hypothesis that caffeine is added not just to increase the liking of soda but also to increase the reinforcing properties of soda. Specifically, she and her research team designed a study aimed at testing whether caffeinated soda becomes reinforcing over time (Temple et al., 2009).

Temple described the study participants as 12 to 17 years of age, stratified by caffeine use (<25 mg/day; 25–50 mg/day; 50–75 mg/day; and >75 mg/day). The researchers set up an operant response condition in the lab, where participants pressed a mouse button and after so many mouse button presses were reinforced with a portion of soda. Participants were provided both caffeinated and noncaffeinated versions of the same soda and were evaluated for their willingness to work for each type of soda. After the test, participants were sent home with four 2-liter bottles of either caffeinated or noncaffeinated soda, with participants not knowing which type they had, where they consumed the same amount of soda daily (32 oz) for 1 week. At the end of the first week, they were interviewed about how they liked the soda and their mood over the course of the week and were then provided with the opposite type of soda (either noncaffeinated or caffeinated) and asked to again consume the same amount of soda daily (32 oz) for another week. At the end of the second week, participants were again interviewed about how they liked the soda and what their mood had been like. They were also evaluated again for their willingness to work for each type of soda.

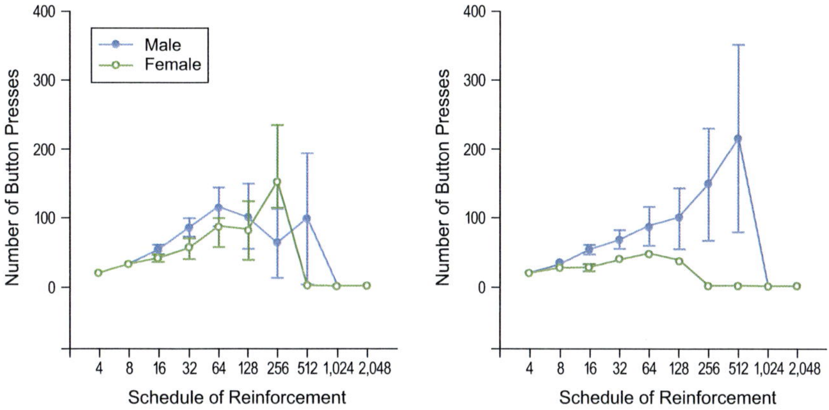

FIGURE 6-1 Results from operant response test for caffeinated soda.
NOTES: Baseline results in the left graph and results obtained after exposure in the right graph. See text for detailed explanation.
SOURCE: Temple et al., 2009.

The results for willingness to work for a caffeinated soda are illustrated in Figure 6-1, with the panel on the left reflecting baseline results and the panel on the right showing results obtained after the exposure period. The y-axis represents the number of button presses; the x-axis represents the number of times the button had to be pressed in order to receive a soda. Typically, data like these show an increase in the number of button presses (y) as the schedule of reinforcement increases (x) and then a decrease. With these data, at baseline, there was no difference between males and females. But after the exposure period, the reinforcement value in males increased significantly, and the reinforcement value in females decreased slightly. That is, after becoming more familiar with caffeinated soda, the soda became more reinforcing for males and less reinforcing for females. Temple did not show the data, but she said that there was no change in the reinforcing value of the noncaffeinated soda in either males or females. Nor were any differences observed on the basis of use (stratification). In sum, according to Temple, the study showed that adding caffeine to soda can increase the reinforcing value of soda.

Next, Temple and her colleagues wanted to see whether caffeine increases subjective liking of soda. Again, they stratified their participants by caffeine use. They provided participants with seven novel sodas on their visit and then picked the beverage ranked fourth by each participant. For each of four subsequent visits, participants were provided with that number four beverage either with or without caffeine (either 1 mg or 2 mg per kg). On the sixth visit, participants were asked to rerate the liking and ranking of that beverage. As described in Temple et al. (2012), individuals in the placebo group did not change their liking of the soda over time. Individuals provided with 1 mg per kg dose of caffeinated soda showed an increase in liking only during the last visit but not before then. Individuals provided with 2 mg per kg showed a steady increase in liking over time. Temple mentioned that similar findings have been observed in adults and with caffeinated yogurt (Panek et al., 2013).

Cardiovascular Response to Caffeine

With respect to cardiovascular effects in children, Temple and colleagues conducted a double-blind, placebo-controlled, dose–response study in which each child (aged 12 to 17 years) was administered one of four doses of caffeine on four different visits and in which his or her heart rate and systolic and diastolic blood pressure were measured (Temple et al., 2010). Both males and females showed a dose-dependent decrease in heart rate and dose-dependent increase in blood pressure. When the researchers compared low and high users, however, they found no difference in females, but among males they found a stronger cardiovascular response among high users. These latter results, together with the results from Temple et al. (2009), suggest to Temple that there might be some gender differences in response to caffeine.

In a subsequent study, Temple and her team conducted the same tests on prepubertal versus postpubertal children. They found that, for both heart rate and systolic blood pressure, postpubertal females show dampened responses to caffeine compared to males. That is, they showed less change in both heart rate and systolic blood pressure. Among prepubertal children, there was no difference between females and males. These results suggest to Temple that the gender difference in caffeine response emerges after puberty.

Subjective Effects of Caffeine

A similar gender difference has also been observed in subjective effects of caffeine. As also described in Temple et al. (2010), Temple and her team used a questionnaire to evaluate study participants’ reasons for using caffeine. The researchers found that males were much more likely to report using caffeine to get energy, to get a rush, and to enhance either academic or athletic performance. They found no difference between males and females in the use of caffeine to concentrate or because friends use caffeine. These findings suggest to Temple that males experience stronger subjective effects of caffeine than females do, at least within the 12- to 17-year-old age range.

In a follow-up study, Temple et al. (2012) looked directly at subjective effects in postpubertal children. The researchers gave questionnaires to participants after administering either a placebo (no caffeine) or 2 mg caffeine per kg. Males reported feeling the effects of caffeine more, liking it more, feeling "high," and wanting more. Females actually showed a negative response to the caffeine. Compared to the placebo, they reported feeling it less, liking it less, feeling less "high," and wanting it less than they wanted the placebo. Again, these results suggest to Temple that there is a gender difference in response to caffeine.

Cognitive Effects of Caffeine

Most recently, Temple and colleagues have been examining the cognitive effects of caffeine in prepubertal versus postpubertal children. Temple described an unpublished study where participants were administered either 0, 1 mg caffeine per kg, or 2 mg caffeine per kg. The researchers tested cognitive response at baseline and again after an hour, using a cognitive battery that could be used in 8- and 9-year-old children as well as in 15- and 16-year-old children (i.e., simple reaction times, complex reaction times, memory search, Stroop, go/no-go). Compared to the placebo (0 caffeine), both the 1 mg of caffeine per kg and the 2 mg of caffeine per kg doses improved the number correct, reaction time, and number correct per minute on the Stroop test and reduced the standard deviation of the Stroop test. In general, according to Temple, caffeine affects cognitive functioning in children. She noted a few subtle effects of gender but did not describe them.

Future Directions

In sum, caffeine definitely has effects in children that are consistent with some findings in adults. The biggest difference, in Temple's opinion, is that there do not seem to be many differences between low versus high caffeine users. In fact, she and her colleagues have not found any significant differences between low versus high caffeine users. Temple attributes the lack of such differences to the fact that even what are considered high users among children are children who still use caffeine relatively infrequently and at relatively smaller doses compared to adults. It is possible that children have not yet developed tolerance for the effects of caffeine.

In the future, Temple said, she would like to understand the relationship between early caffeine use and later drug use. She remarked that there are some good cross-sectional data showing that caffeine enhances the reinforcing value of nicotine in humans (Jones and Griffiths, 2003) and some good experimental data showing that caffeine enhances the reinforcing value of cocaine in rats (Green and Schenk, 2002). Caffeine has also been shown to induce dopamine release in the nucleus accumbens (Acquas et al., 2002) and to condition flavor preferences in adults (Yeomans et al., 2000, 2001; Yeomans, 2004; Panek et al., 2013) and in children (Temple et al., 2012). These findings suggest to Temple that there could be a relationship between caffeine and drug use. She would like to study that relationship in a prospective design where early caffeine use is measured and children are followed over time.

In conclusion, Temple identified several data gaps in the literature. First, while preparing her presentation, she found it very difficult to find a current survey of caffeine use in adults and children in the United States. Many of the data she found were old and did not really capture the potential shifts in usage since energy drinks have flooded the market. In addition to prospective studies on relationships between early caffeine use and later substance use, she called for prospective studies examining factors that relate to high caffeine use and risk of high-level caffeine use. Finally, she called for studies on the long-term effects of caffeine use, particularly studies beginning in childhood and progressing to adulthood.

ADDICTIVE PROPERTIES OF CAFFEINE

Presented by Roland R. Griffiths, Ph.D.,
Johns Hopkins University School of Medicine

Roland Griffiths provided an overview of the evidence for five human behavioral effects of caffeine: subjective effects, reinforcing effects, tolerance, physical dependence (i.e., withdrawal), and addiction.[1]

[1]The American Society for Addictive Medicine defines addiction as "characterized by inability to consistently abstain, impairment in behavioral control, craving, diminished

Subjective Effects

Griffiths described the subjective effects as drug-induced changes in an individual's experience or feelings. Numerous studies have shown that the qualitative subjective effects of caffeine are dose dependent, with lower doses (20–200 mg) producing predominately positive subjective effects, such as well-being, energy, and alertness. Higher doses (300–500 mg) produce predominately dysphoric subjective effects.

Reinforcing Effects

Reinforcing effects, which refer to the self-administration of caffeine, have been demonstrated very clearly in both laboratory animals (e.g., baboons) and humans. Griffiths summarized key findings from approximately 20 scientific studies on reinforcing effects of caffeine in humans:

- Caffeine can function as a reinforcer when administered in capsules, coffee, or soft drinks.
- The range of conditions under which caffeine functions as a reinforcer is not as broad as with classic psychomotor stimulants such as amphetamine or cocaine.
- Caffeine reinforcement is an inverted U-shaped function of dose.
- In normal subjects there are wide individual differences in susceptibility to caffeine reinforcement.
- Avoidance of abstinence-associated withdrawal symptoms plays a central role in reinforcement among regular consumers. Nevertheless, such a history is not necessary for demonstrating caffeine reinforcement.

In addition, there is overwhelming circumstantial evidence that caffeine has reinforcing effects: regular daily consumption of pharmacologically active doses is widespread, with caffeine being the most widely used mood-altering drug in the world; historically, caffeine consumption has been long term, relatively stable, and resistant to suppression; and

---

recognition of significant problems with one's behaviors and interpersonal relationships, and a dysfunctional emotional response." Available at http://www.asam.org/for-the-public/definition-of-addiction (accessed January 13, 2014).

consumption occurs in widely different vehicles and in widely varying cultural and social contexts.

Tolerance

Tolerance, which refers to reduced responsiveness due to drug exposure, has been clearly demonstrated in both laboratory animals and humans. Studies with rats have shown that chronically treated rats show no response to caffeine, compared to untreated rats, who exhibit an inverted U-shaped response. Studies with rats have also shown no cross-tolerance to amphetamine. Complete tolerance also occurs in humans at high doses. For example, Griffiths and colleagues showed that a 300-mg challenge to caffeine-free individuals maintained on placebo caused tension, anxiety, and jitteriness, compared to a total absence of effect among individuals receiving a chronic dose of 900 mg per day (Evans and Griffiths, 1992).

Physical Dependence

Physical dependence, or withdrawal, refers to time-limited disruption of mood or behavior after cessation of chronic dosing. Withdrawal has been very well demonstrated in both animals and humans. Activity in rats has been shown to decrease when switched from chronic caffeine to water, with recovery to normal activity occurring over the course of several days. Similar results have been observed in humans. Griffiths and colleagues demonstrated increased headaches and lethargy and decreased ability to concentrate after abruptly switching individuals from caffeine to placebo, with the effects resolving over the course of several days to a week (Griffiths et al., 1990). In another study in which individuals were blind to the manipulation (Silverman et al., 1992), about 50 percent of individuals who were switched from caffeine to placebo reported moderate or severe headache and about 11 to 12 percent reported substantial increases in depression and fatigue. Individuals switched from caffeine to placebo also demonstrated decreased psychomotor tapping performance and increased unauthorized medication use, mostly for headache. According to Griffiths, in the approximately 75 experimental studies conducted that permit this kind of analysis, about 50 percent of individuals reported headache (Juliano and Griffiths, 2004). So headache is a common symptom of withdrawal, although withdrawal can also occur without headache.

Headache is one of several caffeine withdrawal symptom clusters recognized by the DSM-5. Others are fatigue or drowsiness; dysphoric mood; depressed mood; irritability; difficulty concentrating; and flu-like somatic symptoms (nausea, vomiting, or muscle pain/stiffness). In the literature, the incidence of clinically significant or functional impairment (i.e., people unable to do what they normally do) averages 13 percent in prospective experimental studies and 9 percent in retrospective survey studies (Juliano and Griffiths, 2004). As just one example, Griffiths mentioned the range of functional impairments reported in a double-blind placebo-controlled challenge study: missed work and vomited; could not perform work responsibilities, needed spouse to care for children, and went to bed early; performed multiple costly mistakes at work, left work early, and went to bed early; screamed at children (Strain et al., 1994).

A variety of studies have shown caffeine withdrawal to be what Griffiths described as "a robust parametric phenomenon." Chronic maintenance dose, duration of caffeine maintenance, and within-day frequency of dosing all impact the probability and severity of withdrawal. Even just three days of chronic exposure and once-a-day administration are sufficient to trigger withdrawal signals. In addition, readministration of caffeine has been shown to reverse abstinence effects in a very rapid and dose-dependent way.

Equally important, in Griffiths's opinion, many studies have demonstrated that avoidance of abstinence-associated withdrawal symptoms plays a central role in the habitual consumption of caffeine. Studies have also demonstrated that withdrawal potentiates the reinforcing effects of caffeine and that withdrawal plays an important role in the development of preferences for flavors paired with caffeine (Juliano and Griffiths, 2004). Regarding the latter point, Griffiths referred workshop participants to some of the data cited by Jennifer Temple during her presentation.

Addiction: DSM Substance Dependence Syndrome

The DSM-5 does not officially recognize caffeine addiction, or dependence syndrome, as a diagnosis, given that too few studies have been completed; they did propose research criteria. Still, Griffiths identified eight studies showing that some people do in fact fulfill DSM-4 or DSM-5 criteria for a diagnosis of substance dependence as applied to caffeine: Strain et al. (1994), Hughes et al. (1998), Bernstein et al. (2002), Jones and Lejuez (2005), Svikis et al. (2005), Ciapparelli et al. (2010), Striley et al. (2011), and Juliano et al. (2012).

For example, in a study of individuals who were sufficiently distressed by their caffeine use to seek outpatient treatment, Juliano et al. (2012) evaluated what they identified as the three DSM-5 criteria most definitional of addiction. Individuals were recruited from the community using advertisements inviting participation in a program for caffeine dependence. In an effort to be very conservative and include only hard cases of pure caffeine dependence, individuals with other current drug dependence excepting nicotine were excluded. The group comprised 94 total participants. Griffiths described them as a high-functioning educated group of adults. Their mean age was 41 years, 55 percent were female, and 86 percent were college or postgraduate educated. Mean caffeine use was 548 mg/day, so it was over the 90th percentile. A clinical psychologist conducted the evaluations.

Among the 94 total participants in Juliano et al. (2012), 89 percent reported persistent desire or unsuccessful efforts to cut down or control substance use; 96 percent reported characteristic withdrawal symptoms or use to relieve or avoid withdrawal symptoms, with 43 percent reporting functional impairment (i.e., severity sufficient to produce an impairment of normal activities, such as being unable to work or sleeping at work); 87 percent reported continued use despite persistent or recurrent physical or psychological problems. Regarding the reports of physical or psychological problems, 83 percent reported physical problems (e.g., stomach problems, cardiovascular problems, complications of pregnancy, sleep problems, urinary problems); 67 percent reported psychological problems (e.g., anxiety, irritability, anger); and 43 percent reported having been told by a physician or other medical professional to modify their caffeine use because of various medical conditions (e.g., pregnancy, headache).

Conclusions with Respect to Caffeine Withdrawal and Addiction

In Griffiths's opinion, with respect to withdrawal, numerous studies, around 75 percent, indicate that cessation of caffeine consumption after a period of daily intake can result in a distressing withdrawal syndrome involving functional impairment. This conclusion is consistent with the DSM-5 committee recognition of caffeine withdrawal as a diagnosis. It is also consistent with a recent survey of 500 addiction professionals—

most of whom endorsed the idea that caffeine withdrawal can be of clinical importance (Budney et al., 2013).

Caffeine addiction is a less well-established effect than caffeine withdrawal, which is consistent with the DSM-5 committee recommendation that caffeine use disorder be recommended as a diagnosis for further study. Still, Griffiths pointed out that the majority of addiction professionals surveyed in Budney et al. (2013) endorsed the idea that caffeine use disorder occurs and that some people could benefit from professional help in quitting. Griffiths identified eight studies suggesting that some people become clinically dependent on caffeine, that is, they are unable to quit, they continue to use despite medical problems, and they are sufficiently distressed to seek treatment (Meredith et al., 2013).

Implications for Youth as a Vulnerable Population

Several of these findings have potential implications for youth. First, with respect to tolerance, Griffiths said, individuals who do not use caffeine regularly will likely be substantially more sensitive to the acute effects of caffeine, including its adverse effects. Studies show that tolerance readily occurs, with lower doses leading to partial tolerance and higher doses to complete and insurmountable tolerance. Nevertheless, because most studies characterizing the adverse effects of caffeine have examined those effects in habitual consumers, they are of little relevance in estimating the risk of adverse events in nonusers.

Another implication for youth is that caffeine reinforcement, tolerance, and withdrawal are dose dependent. Individuals who weigh less receive a proportionally greater dose of caffeine for a given serving size, with a 13-year-old boy weighing about 55 percent as much as a 50-year-old man.

Conditioned taste preference also has implications for youth as a vulnerable population. It is well known that consumers often develop strong preferences for specific types and brands of caffeinated beverages. The likely mechanism behind this is that caffeine conditions specific flavor preferences, with initial flavor preferences likely evolving into habitual brand preferences, perhaps lasting a lifetime. Griffiths opined that these facts are not lost on those marketing energy drinks and may incentivize promotion of products to younger and younger populations, much as the tobacco companies were accused of doing until such marketing became more tightly regulated.

Finally, Griffiths noted, with respect to withdrawal and addiction, if physical dependence develops, youth are less likely to have the financial, transportation, or other resources to ensure an uninterrupted supply of caffeine. When their habitual pattern of intake is delayed or disrupted, withdrawal-sensitive individuals experience adverse emotional, cognitive, and behavioral consequences.

DSM-5: SUBSTANCE-RELATED AND ADDICTION DISORDERS

Presented by Charles P. O'Brien, M.D., Ph.D.,
University of Pennsylvania, Philadelphia

Charles O'Brien emphasized that addictive disorders are a complex area of study because of individual variation, including the role of genetics in drug reactivity. He suggested that a genetic factor may explain why some people develop what is now being called caffeine use disorder (i.e., caffeine addiction) and others do not.

Substance Use Disorder: Differences Between DSM-IV and DSM-5

O'Brien served for 7 years as chair of the DSM-5[2] committee, and he explained some important differences between the DSM-IV and DSM-5. First, for all drugs, the DSM-IV differentiated between use, abuse, and addiction. On reexamining 150,000 diagnostic interviews, the DSM-5 committee realized that the severity of use is a progressive phenomenon, from gradual use to addiction. The DSM-5 committee identified 11 symptoms, with a greater number of symptoms indicating greater severity: tolerance (not counted if prescribed by a physician); withdrawal (not counted if prescribed by a physician); more use than intended; craving for the substance; unsuccessful efforts to cut down; excessive time spent in acquisition; activities given up because of use; use despite negative effects; failure to fulfill major role obligations; recurrent use in hazardous situations; and continued use despite consistent social or interpersonal problems. Generally, exhibiting two symptoms is considered mild, up

---

[2]As O'Brien explained, the DSM, the major classification of mental illness, is used worldwide; the DSM-5 was published in May 2012 and is the current official version.

to four is moderate, and over four is severe. All but one of the 11 symptoms were recognized in DSM-IV. The DSM-5 committee eliminated liver problems as a symptom because it was considered not useful, and they added craving. O'Brien described tolerance as a "normal reaction," with caffeine being one of several types of drugs that shows very rapid tolerance. Others are antihypertensive drugs, antidepressants, antianxiety drugs, and opioid analgesics.

The DSM-5 committee did not include addiction, or caffeine use disorder, as a diagnosis. But they did include it in the appendix to stimulate research. O'Brien said, "Most of us are not prepared to say that there is such a thing as caffeine addiction, but there is definitely caffeine withdrawal." According to O'Brien, many committee members resisted adding caffeine withdrawal disorder to DSM-5. But for the committee, it was a trivial issue. The evidence is abundant that caffeine withdrawal exists, ranging from very mild to very severe.

A Double-Blind Controlled Study of Caffeine Withdrawal

Impressed with the many placebo-controlled studies they had each conducted over the course of their careers, with individuals in placebo groups reporting many of the same adverse effects reported by individuals in treatment groups, from headache to psychosis, O'Brien and colleague Peter Dews were curious about the "real effects" of caffeine withdrawal. As far as O'Brien was aware, the study they conducted to answer that question, Dews et al. (1999), is the only study of its type where at no point during the study did the researchers tell the participants that they were studying caffeine withdrawal. Starting with a population of about 11,000 people, some of whom consumed caffeinated beverages on a daily basis, the researchers asked participants about problems with stopping caffeine and randomized participants who reported withdrawal into three groups. All three groups received roughly the same 400–500 mg daily dose of caffeine for 1 week to 10 days. After the 10-day period of stabilization, one group continued to receive the same dose, the second group experienced abrupt withdrawal, and the third group received a gradual reduction in dose. Then the researchers asked participants a series of questions about their energy, alertness, leisure time, and other symptoms. To distract participants, the researchers also asked about the smell, appearance, and taste of coffee (i.e., those questions were considered a distracter because the researchers were interested only in withdrawal). The end result was that individuals who continued to receive the same dose showed no withdrawal symptoms; females in the sudden reduction group showed symptoms—for example, they reported being less alert—but males showed no symptoms; and individuals in the gradual withdrawal group reported minimal if any symptoms. According to O'Brien, withdrawal may not be as common as placebo-controlled studies suggest.

ENERGY DRINK USE AND RISK TAKING DURING ADOLESCENCE AND YOUNG ADULTHOOD

Presented by Amelia Arria, Ph.D.,
University of Maryland, College Park

At an FDA public hearing on functional foods on December 5, 2006, Amelia Arria and colleagues submitted remarks on the association between the consumption of highly caffeinated energy drinks and risk-taking behavior. At this IOM workshop, Arria discussed additional evidence that has accumulated since that time and that has raised concerns among public health professionals worldwide about the possible contribution of energy drink consumption to risk-taking behavior that ultimately impacts the health and safety of adolescents and young adults. Specifically, she presented new research in the field of developmental neuroscience that has shed light on the complex changes that take place in the brain during adolescence. She also shared evidence from her own prospective research showing that high levels of caffeine in the new ways that caffeine is being consumed and in the new products now available might exacerbate the health risk-taking behavior of adolescents.

Neurodevelopmental Influences on Risk-Taking Behavior During Adolescence

Scientists have learned a great deal during the past 20 years, especially the past 10 years, about the human brain and how the brain undergoes very complex and functional changes during the adolescent years and into the early 20s (Kuhn, 2006; Crews et al., 2007; Steinberg, 2008; Johnson et al., 2009; White, 2009; Casey and Jones, 2010; Gladwin et al., 2011; Pharo et al., 2011; Sturman and Mogghaddam, 2011; Spear, 2013). These changes partially explain why adolescents are more likely than older individuals to engage in risk-taking behavior and perhaps less likely to fully recognize the consequences of such behavior. Moreover, adolescents appear to be more susceptible to the rewarding properties of substances. The evidence also helps to explain the long-established robust finding that early use of substances increases the risk of addiction in adulthood. In short, Arria explained, there is an inherent vulnerability of the developing brain to psychoactive substances.

Energy Drinks: Potential Exacerbation of Health-Risk Behaviors

Several naturalistic and one experimental study have clearly demonstrated that energy drink users are more likely to engage in risk-taking behavior (Miller, 2008; Arria et al., 2010, 2011; Stasio et al., 2011; Velaquez et al., 2012; Peacock et al., 2013; Woolsey et al., 2013). Many forms of risk-taking behavior have been studied, including drug use, sexual risk taking, alcohol use, and the mixing of energy drinks and alcohol. Arria also considers studies on anxiety and sleep quality important factors to consider when evaluating adolescent behavior, even though they are not necessarily considered risk-taking behaviors. The one experimental study, Peacock et al. (2013), involved measuring risk-taking behavior in a laboratory setting using an analog measure called BART (Balloon Analogue Risk Task).

Arria noted that the frequency of energy drink use among the studies she was able to locate that specifically focused on risk-taking behavior were studies on college students and that the prevalence estimates of energy drink consumption among that age group are much higher than was alluded to earlier during the workshop discussion. Recent studies are showing prevalence estimates of up to 83 percent in the past year and 57 percent in the past week (i.e., the year or week prior to collecting data). Her research team's data have shown a 65 percent annual increase in prevalence of use between the second and third years of college. She suggested that snapshot measures of 2-day or 7-day frequency cannot capture past year or past month use and identified the lack of valid assessment methods for energy drink consumption as an important data gap.

According to Arria, contrary to an earlier workshop remark that there are no prospective data on the relationship between energy drink use and subsequent use of other drugs, she and her colleagues have in fact been collecting prospective data on a cohort of more than 1,200 students, with a response rate of 81 percent. The study is now in its 10th year. The researchers have examined the relationship between different types of substances and the subsequent increase in the use of other substances over time. As far as she knows, the data represent the only prospective epidemiologic data on energy drink consumption over time in a large sample of young adults. Specifically, guided by prior research suggesting that caffeine use might exacerbate the underlying vulnerability to the use of other substances, the researchers asked whether energy drink use during the second year of college predicted incident or new use of other drugs during the following year.

After adjusting for sex, demographics, socioeconomic status, sensation seeking (i.e., according to Arria, a variable that measures novelty seeking), and other types of caffeine use, the researchers found that, yes, the use of energy drinks in the second year of college (23 percent of the sample) predicted frequency of tobacco use and incident (new) nonmedical use of prescription stimulants and prescription analgesics in the third year (Arria et al., 2010). The adjusted odds ratio for stimulants was 2.5 ($p < 0.001$), with 8.2 percent of nonenergy drink users and 18.8 percent of energy drink users starting to use prescription stimulants the following year (see Figure 6-2). The adjusted odds ratio for analgesics was 1.5 ($p < 0.05$).

Implications of This New Evidence

In Arria's opinion, new evidence from developmental neuroscience underscores the inherent vulnerability of the developing brain to psychoactive substances. In addition, the balance of evidence in the scientific literature supports the argument that the levels of caffeine in today's products, in the way those products are consumed, are associated with increased risk-taking behaviors. Nor has the addition of caffeine to energy drinks at the levels present in most products been demonstrated to be safe with regard to risk-taking behaviors in adolescents and young adults. Until evidence has been presented that demonstrates safety, actions to change current regulations on these products are warranted to protect and promote the health of the public in general and the health of adolescents in particular.

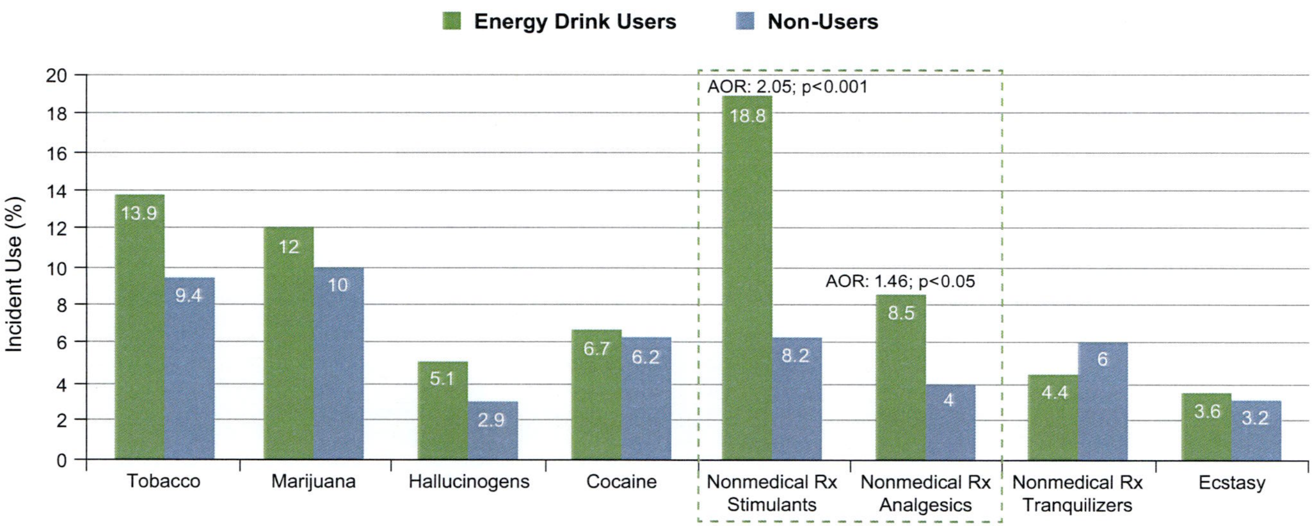

FIGURE 6-2 Summary of results from prospective study on energy drink use among second-year college students and the use of other substances during the third year of college.
NOTE: AOR = adjusted odds ratio.
SOURCE: Arria et al., 2010.

CAFFEINE, PERFORMANCE, AND WELL-BEING

Presented by Andrew P. Smith, Ph.D.,
Cardiff University, UK

During the "caffeine wars" of the 1990s, while experts debated the health effects of caffeine exposure, according to Andrew Smith, they also acknowledged that there were some areas, such as cognitive psychology, where one could actually demonstrate benefits of caffeine exposure. A typical finding was that reaction time scores measured 60 minutes after ingesting caffeine improved when tested in a double-blind, placebo-controlled trial, with the caffeinated group showing faster reaction times than the noncaffeinated group (see Figure 6-3). Another well-established finding was that the number of targets detected in a sustained attention task increased with increasing caffeine dose (see Figure 6-3).

One of the areas where the benefits of caffeine have been most easily demonstrated is in low-alertness situations—for example, when people are working at night. The reaction time among people working at night slows quite dramatically over the course of a night, with caffeine improving reaction time and with the difference in reaction time between caffeinated and decaffeinated conditions becoming greater over the course of a night. Other low-alertness situations where caffeine may be beneficial include after lunch, when people are sick with minor illnesses such as colds, and when people are fatigued because of prolonged work.

These and other findings led the European Food Safety Authority (EFSA) in 2011 to conclude that "a cause and effect relationship has been established between the consumption of caffeine and increased attention" said Smith. The EFSA further established that in order to bear the claim, a product should contain 75 mg of caffeine. According to Smith, the EFSA decision was applicable only to adults. There were some concerns about children consuming those doses.

Another area where caffeine has been shown to be especially beneficial is in removing the effects of sleep deprivation. In 2005 the American Academy of Sleep Medicine reviewed the evidence and concluded that 14 of 15 studies showed increased wakefulness following ingestion of caffeine by sleep-deprived volunteers.

In sum, according to Smith, there are some very well established beneficial effects of caffeine. There are also some very plausible mechanisms to explain the beneficial effects of caffeine. Smith mentioned two.

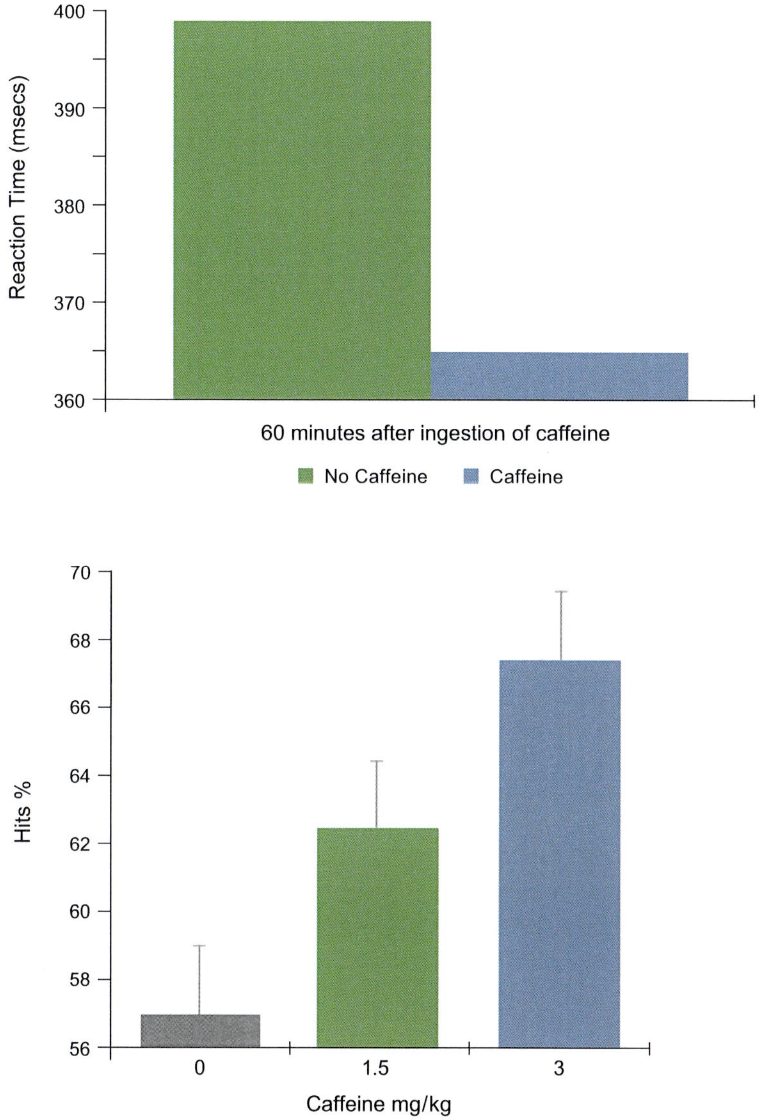

FIGURE 6-3 Typical findings reported in the 1990s. Reaction time as a function of caffeine exposure (top) and number of targets detected in a sustained attention task as a function of caffeine dose (bottom).
SOURCES: Smith et al., 1993; Brice and Smith, 2001.

First, he and colleagues have shown that the effects of caffeine in low-alertness situations reflect changes in central noradrenaline. Smith acknowledged the earlier workshop discussion on the effects of caffeine on dopamine (see Ferré's summary at the beginning of this chapter), but he noted that, in terms of changes in cognition and alertness, other neurotransmitters, such as noradrenalin, are also very important. Typical studies of the effect of caffeine on noradrenalin rely on the drug clonidine, which reduces the turnover of noradrenalin and creates a state very similar to sleep deprivation. Not surprisingly, Smith observed, when people are administered clonidine, they react more slowly than people administered a placebo. When the clonidine is combined with caffeine, however, the caffeine restores function to a level not significantly different from that of the control group.

Cholinergic changes are another plausible mechanism to explain the beneficial effects of caffeine, one that does not depend on alertness being low. According to Smith, caffeine has been shown to improve the speed of encoding new information via cholinergic changes, with reaction time to new stimuli decreasing as the caffeine dose increases.

Practical Implications

According to Smith, the study that arguably demonstrates most clearly the practical implications of all these various findings on the beneficial effects of caffeine exposure is Lieberman et al.'s (2002) study on caffeine and sustained military operations. The researchers examined the effects of caffeine in U.S. Navy Seals during what is known as "hell week," a very fatiguing and stressful training week where the Seals conduct excessive work on little sleep. The researchers found that a dose of 200 mg of caffeine improved vigilance, learning, memory, and mood and concluded that the administration of caffeine may provide a significant advantage when cognitive performance is critical and must be maintained during exposure to severe stress.

Smith himself has examined the impact of caffeine on real-life work performance in two ways. The first was what Smith described as an "after-effect" technique, which involves obtaining both subjective and objective measurements both before and after work and using the difference between the before- and after-work measurements as an indicator of performance during the work period. So someone who had a very fatiguing work day would show a much larger after-effect of that day compared to someone who had a relatively light work day. Smith (2005) measured reported alertness and simple reaction time among 110 workers both before and after work and found that workers who had consumed caffeine during the day were more alert and had faster reaction times.

Because after-effect measures are only indirect measures of work performance, Smith has also conducted epidemiological research on associations between caffeine consumption and accidents or errors during work. Specifically, Smith (2005) sampled more than 2,500 workers who were in jobs where accident risk was high and found that higher caffeine consumption was associated with half the risk of frequent cognitive failures and accidents. (Cognitive failures are human errors involving problems with memory and attention.)

An Alternative View?

Although these findings tell what Smith said is a "very nice story," he acknowledged that there is an alternative view: that caffeine has no positive effects, that rather it just removes the negative effects of caffeine withdrawal. He referred to earlier workshop discussions on the negative effects of caffeine withdrawal, including headaches, mood changes, and impaired performance (see summaries of Roland Griffiths's and Charles O'Brien's presentations earlier in this chapter). In Smith's opinion, this alternative view is unlikely for three reasons. First, the same (beneficial) effects can be observed in animals and in nonconsumers who by definition cannot be withdrawing. Second, the effects are observed even with repeated doses. If the withdrawal explanation were correct, then one would observe effects after the first dose but not after repeated doses. Third, the effects are observed following "wash-out," that is, 1 week to 10 days after withdrawal when negative withdrawal effects are no longer present. Again, if the withdrawal explanation were correct, one should not see effects after withdrawal is over.

In addition, said Smith, effects are observed between different personality types (e.g., introverts versus extroverts) even with the same level of withdrawal. Again, the reversal of withdrawal is an unlikely explanation for these differences. The differences are more likely caused by arousal effects. Also, acute cardiovascular effects of caffeine and the effects of caffeine on sleep are usually explained in terms of stimulant effects. It is not clear why another mechanism, that is, withdrawal reversal, is needed to explain such effects.

Conclusions About Caffeine and Performance

In conclusion, Smith reiterated that the levels of caffeine consumed by most people have largely beneficial effects on alertness, attention, and other similar behaviors. He emphasized, however, that excessive consumption can lead to problems, especially in sensitive individuals. For Smith, here "sensitive" means a child. In a pilot study on diet, behavior, and attainment in 200 secondary school children, researchers found several associations between diet and detention (personal communication, Nicholas Milward, Pool Academy, January 2012). For example, students who consumed energy drinks were 60 percent more likely to receive detention.

On the basis of the results of that pilot study, Smith and colleagues conducted a longitudinal study involving 2,000 pupils. They administered two dietary surveys, one at the start and the other at the end of the school year, and collected two sets of measures of attainment and behavior. The researchers are currently analyzing cross-sectional data.[3] Thus far, they have shown that those who often consumed energy drinks were more likely to have low attendance, receive a sanction, and receive poorer grades. These findings are true even when controlling for possible confounders, such as socioeconomic status and special educational needs.

Smith acknowledged that he and his colleagues are unable to infer causality. Longitudinal data and dose–response data will provide a clearer view, as will results of a planned intervention study aimed at measuring the effects of reducing energy drink intake. Until such clarity is reached, there are two plausible mechanisms. Either energy drinks are causing the problems among the school children that he and his colleagues are observing, or energy drink consumption may itself be an outcome, with some other factor driving both energy drink consumption and poor attainment, attendance, and behavior. It is a critical distinction, Smith observed, and one that they hope to have an initial answer for soon.

PANELIST DISCUSSION WITH THE AUDIENCE

This section provides a synopsis of the panelist discussions that took place after the sessions summarized in this chapter. Most of the questions

---

[3]Smith, A. P. 2012–2014. Effects of energy drinks and junk food on school children. Project funded by the Waterloo Foundation.

asked of the panelists revolved around data they had presented, including how those data are being interpreted and gaps in data.

Mechanism of Caffeine's Effect on the Central Nervous System

There was some discussion about conflicting results in the scientific literature on where exactly dopamine is released after exposure to caffeine. Ferré explained that as he mentioned during his talk, caffeine is a weak "dopamine releaser" (although more research needs to be done on the clear dopamine-releasing properties of paraxanthine). Nevertheless, he and his research team found that caffeine in fact induces dopamine release in a specific part of the shell of the nucleus accumbens and that other data suggesting that it occurs not in the nucleus accumbens but in the cortex might be the result of contamination from the shell of the accumbens. He referred workshop participants to a review that he and his team wrote explaining the difference (Ferré, 2008). The take-home message, according to Ferré, is that caffeine is not a very good dopamine releaser when compared to cocaine or amphetamine, because the main mechanism is postsynaptic and results from adenosine-dopamine receptor interactions.

When asked how to reconcile the fact that the mechanism of action for caffeine (which acts on adenosine receptors) is very different from the mechanism of action for cocaine (which acts on dopamine receptors), Ferré responded that the effects are similar because they act in the same brain areas, that is, in the striatum, and that the difference is more quantitative than qualitative.

Most of the panel discussion following Arria's presentation revolved around the interpretation of the evidence presented and the gaps in data.

Cross-Sectional Versus Prospective Studies for Evaluating Long-Term Effects of Exposure in Children

There was a question about the roles of cross-sectional versus prospective designs in evaluating the long-term effects of caffeine exposure in children and adolescents. Temple remarked that cross-sectional data are confounded in many ways and that there is a strong need for long-term prospective studies.

Cardiovascular Effects of Caffeine Exposure in Children and Adolescents: Sex Differences

Temple was asked whether any of her research involved electrocardiogram monitoring of children and adolescents. Temple explained that her team was not set up to do that and agreed that it would be interesting. Her team measured only heart rate and blood pressure. In this regard, John Higgins expressed intrigue at the blood pressure findings described by Temple, specifically the sex difference found after puberty and the greater responsiveness seen in postpubertal males in comparison to postpubertal females to some of the effects of caffeine. He noted that five of the six deaths reported to be associated with caffeine-containing energy beverages were in males between the ages of 12 and 19. Temple suggested that the difference might be related to circulating steroid hormones. According to Temple, it is well known that steroid hormones affect caffeine metabolism. She and her team are trying to figure out how to test that hypothesis other than by measuring salivary hormone levels. Other data (which she did not present) have shown that blood pressure effects in females are lower when salivary estradiol levels are higher. Temple reiterated that she and her research team have found a greater responsiveness to caffeine among postpubertal males "across the board," that is, not just with cardiovascular effects but also with reinforcing and subjective effects.

Blinded Studies of Caffeine Withdrawal

Griffiths identified Silverman et al. (1992) as another study on caffeine withdrawal that did not inform participants that caffeine was being tested. Other withdrawal studies have similarly blinded participants (see Juliano and Griffiths, 2004). In Silverman et al. (1992), participants were told only that they were participating in a study on dietary substances. They were provided with misinformation about shellfish, NutraSweet, and so forth, to distract them. In addition, Juliano and Griffiths (2004) have estimated a 13 percent incidence of significant functional impairment, compared to Dews et al.'s (1999) 2.6 percent. Even 2.6 percent is not trivial in a population in which caffeine is consumed by 85 percent of the population, in Griffiths's opinion.

The Association Between Caffeine Use and Other Substance Use in Adolescents and Young Adults

A driver for both caffeine use and the nonmedical use of prescription drugs is the availability of resources needed to acquire those substances, according to a member of the audience. The audience member asked Arria if she and her colleagues had examined the purchasing power of the study participants in the Arria et al. (2010) study and whether possibly the individuals with the ability to purchase caffeinated beverages were, coincidentally, the same individuals with the ability to acquire prescription drugs. Arria explained that she and her team have studied availability and access to nonmedical use of prescription stimulants and have found that, by and large, students obtain them for free from friends, relatives, and acquaintances. The substances are widely accessible. Because all the study participants in Arria et al. (2010) came from the same campus, she thinks it unlikely that some students would have greater access than others.

Arria was also asked about the pattern of use among the students she and her colleagues followed. For example, were they consuming greater doses of energy drinks over time in order to get the same buzz? Were they later substituting analgesics or other substances for the energy drinks because they were no longer getting the same buzz with the energy drinks? Were they using both simultaneously? Arria found it an interesting suggestion that consumption might be related to the likelihood to try something with greater potency. Arria referred workshop participants to a recent study, Woolsey et al. (2013), where the researchers found a great overlap between the substitution of energy drinks and the use of nonmedical prescription stimulants for studying. In addition, the researchers reported that every individual with a prescribed attention deficit hyperactivity disorder (ADHD) medication was using energy drinks, a finding that suggested to Arria that someone should probably be studying the interaction between energy drinks and medical use of prescription stimulants.

Another audience member observed that many people with ADHD self-medicate with caffeine. He asked Arria whether individuals in her study might be substituting the stimulants for caffeine, not necessarily because they were seeking something with greater potency, but as a way to self-medicate. She explained that her study has collected data on the motives of energy drink consumption and has yet to analyze the data.

Arria was also asked whether results were different between female and male participants. She explained that she and her research team controlled for gender in Arria et al. (2010). She noted that she has observed a difference in energy drink use, with a higher proportion of girls drinking coffee and a higher proportion of boys drinking energy drinks.

She was also asked about the nature of the survey. She did not send the survey out to students. Rather, her research team conducted face-to-face interviews. She also clarified that other studies have looked at a variety of risk-taking behaviors but that, for the sake of time, she chose to focus her presentation of the subsequent use of an illicit drug as the behavior of interest. When asked whether she was suggesting that energy drinks were causative of risk-taking behavior, she replied that it will take an accumulation of evidence to infer causality. Arria et al. (2010) was the first of what she hopes will be a series of prospective investigations into the contribution of energy drinks to future illicit drug use. In her opinion, at this point, rather than causality, the focus should be on safety. She said, "I think the burden of proof on whether or not regulations need to occur is really [on] a demonstration of safety rather than on a demonstration of causality." When the same audience member pressed her further about whether there has been a demonstration of causality between energy drinks and risk-taking behavior, she replied that there are very compelling, consistent data across studies to demonstrate a contributory association but agreed that more data are needed to demonstrate causality. When asked about what her theory was, she referred to her earlier comments about neural development of the adolescent brain.

Withdrawal Suppression

Following Smith's presentation, Roland Griffiths commented about withdrawal suppression and the fact that some experts attribute all observed beneficial effects to caffeine withdrawal suppression. "That seems radical," Griffiths said. At the same time, he did not think that the withdrawal suppression hypothesis should be so readily dismissed. The right methodology for addressing it would be a balanced design involving chronic caffeine administration compared to chronic placebo administration (e.g., Sigmon et al., 2009). Smith agreed that the hypothesis should not be dismissed and that there certainly are individuals for whom withdrawal is a significant problem. At the same time, he does not think it is a ubiquitous explanation. He agreed that more research along the lines of what Griffiths suggested is necessary and observed that withdrawal is likely more important with mood changes than with performance changes.

REFERENCES

Acquas, E., G. Tanda, and G. Di Chiara. 2002. Differential effects of caffeine on dopamine and acetylcholine transmission in brain areas of drug-naive and caffeine-pretreated rats. *Neuropsychopharmacology* 27(2):182–193.

Arria, A. M., K. M. Caldeira, S. J. Kasperski, K. E. O'Grady, K. B. Vincent, R. R. Griffiths, and E. D. Wish. 2010. Increased alcohol consumption, nonmedical prescription drug use, and illicit drug use associated with energy drink consumption among college students. *Journal of Addiction Medicine* 4:74–80.

Arria, A. M., K. M. Caldeira, S. J. Kasperski, K. B. Vincent, R. R. Griffiths, and K. E. O'Grady. 2011. Energy drink consumption and increased risk for alcohol dependence. *Alcoholism: Clinical and Experimental Research* 35(2):365–375.

Azdad, K., D. Gall, A. S. Woods, C. Ledent, S. Ferré, and S. N. Schiffmann. 2009. Dopamine D2 and adenosine A2A receptors regulate NMDA-mediated excitation in accumbens neurons through A2A-D2 receptor heteromerization. *Neuropsychopharmacology* 34:972–986.

Bender, A. M., R. L. Donnerstein, R. A. Samson, D. Zhu, and S. J. Goldberg. 1997. Hemodynamic effects of acute caffeine ingestion in young adults. *American Journal of Cardiology* 79(5):696–699.

Bernstein, G. A., M. E. Carroll, P. D. Thuras, K. P. Cosgrove, and M. E. Roth. 2002. Caffeine dependence in teenagers. *Drug and Alcohol Dependence* 66:1–6.

Brice, C. F., and A. P. Smith. 2001. Caffeine levels in saliva: Associations with psychosocial factors and behavioural effects. *Human Psychopharmacology* 16:507–521.

Budney, A. J., P. C. Brown, R. R. Griffiths, J. R. Hughes, and L. M. Juliano. 2013. Caffeine withdrawal and dependence: A convenience survey among addiction professionals. *Journal of Caffeine Research* 3:67–71.

Canals, M., D. Marcellino, F. Fanellis, F. Ciruela, P. de Benedetti, S. R. Goldberg, K. Neve, K. Fuxe, L. F. Agnati, A. S. Woods, S. Ferré, C. Lluis, M. Bouvier, and R. Franco. 2003. Adenosine A2A-dopamine D2 receptor-receptor heteromerization: Qualitative and quantitative assessment by fluorescence and bioluminescence energy transfer. *Journal of Biological Chemistry* 278:46741–46749.

Casey, B. J., and R. M. Jones. 2010. Neurobiology of the adolescent brain and behavior: Implications for substance use disorders. *Journal of American Academy of Child and Adolescent Psychiatry* 49:1189–1201.

Ciapparelli, A., R. Paggini, C. Carmassi, C. Taponecco, G. Consoli, G. Ciampa, C. E. Ramacciotti, D. Marazziti, and L. Dell'Osso. 2010. Patterns of caffeine consumption in psychiatric patients: An Italian study. *European Psychiatry* 25:230–235.

Crews, F., J. He, and C. Hodge. 2007. Adolescent cortical development: A critical period of vulnerability for addiction. *Pharmacology, Biochemistry, and Behavior* 86:189–199.

Davis, J. K., and J. M. Green. 2009. Caffeine and anaerobic performance: Ergogenic value and mechanisms of action. *Sports Medicine* 39(10):813–832.

Dews, P. B., G. L. Curtis, K. J. Hanford, and C. P. O'Brien. 1999. The frequency of caffeine withdrawal in a population-based survey and in a controlled, blinded pilot experiment. *Journal of Clinical Pharmacology* 39(12):1221–1232.

Evans, S. M., and R. R. Griffiths. 1992. Caffeine tolerance and choice in humans. *Psychopharmacology* 108:51–59.

Ferré, S. 2008. An update on the mechanisms of the psychostimulant effects of caffeine. *Journal of Neurochemistry* 105:1067–1079.

Ferré, S. 2010. Role of the central ascending neurotransmitter systems in the psychostimulant effects of caffeine. *Journal of Alzheimer's Disease* 20:S35–S49.

Ferré, S., M. Herrera-Marschitz, M. Grabowska-Andén, U. Ungerstedt, M. Casas, and N. E. Andén. 1991a. Postsynaptic dopamine/adenosine interaction: I. Adenosine analogues inhibit dopamine D2-mediated behavior in short-term reserpinized mice. *European Journal of Pharmacology* 192:25–30.

Ferré, S., A. Rubio, and K. Fuxe. 1991b. Stimulation of adenosine A2 receptors induces catalepsy. *Neuroscience Letters* 130:162–164.

Ferré, S., G. von Euler, B. Johansson, B. B. Fredholm, and K. Fuxe. 1991c. Stimulation of high-affinity adenosine A2 receptors decreases the affinity of dopamine D2 receptors in rat striatal membranes. *Proceedings of the National Academy of Sciences of the United States of America* 88:7238–7241.

Ferré, S., W. T. O'Connor, K. Fuxe, and U. Ungerstedt. 1993. The striopallidal neuron: A main locus for adenosine-dopamine interactions in the brain. *Journal of Neuroscience* 13:5402–5406.

Ferré, S., W. T. O'Connor, P. Svenningsson, L. Bjorklund, J. Lindberg, B. Tinner, I. Stromberg, M. Goldstein, S. O. Ogren, U. Ungerstedt, B. B. Fredholm, and K. Fuxe. 1996. Dopamine D1 receptor-mediated facilitation of GABAergic neurotransmission in the rat strioentopenduncular pathway and its modulation by adenosine A1 receptor-mediated mechanisms. *European Journal of Neuroscience* 8:1545–1553.

Ferré, S., L. F. Agnati, F. Ciruela, C. Lluis, A. S. Woods, K. Fuxe, and R. Franco. 2007. Neurotransmitter receptor heteromers and their integrative role in "local modules": The striatal spine module. *Brain Research Reviews* 55:55–67.

Ferré, S., R. Baler, M. Bouvier, M. G. Caron, L. A. Devi, T. Durroux, K. Fuxe, S. R. George, J. A. Javitch, M. J. Lohse, K. Mackie, G. Milligan, K. D. Pleger, J. P. Pin, N. D. Volkow, M. Waldhoer, A. S. Woods, and R. Franco. 2009. Building a new conceptual framework for receptor heteromers. *Nature Chemical Biology* 5:131–134

Ferré, S., M. Orrú, and X. Guitart. 2013. Paraxanthine: Connecting caffeine to nitric oxide neurotransmission. *Journal of Caffeine Research* 3:72–78.

Frary, C. D., R. K. Johnson, and M. Q. Wang. 2005. Food sources and intakes of caffeine in the diets of persons in the United States. *Journal of the American Dietetic Association* 105:110–113.

Fredholm, B. B., K. Bättig, J. Holmén, A. Nehlig, and E. E. Zvartau . 1999. Actions of caffeine in the brain with special reference to factors that contribute to its widespread use. *Pharmacology Review* 51(1):83–133.

Garrett, B. E., and R. R. Griffiths. 1998. Physical dependence increases the relative reinforcing effects of caffeine versus placebo. *Psychopharmacology* 139(3):195–202.

Gladwin, T. E., B. Figner, E. A. Crone, and R. W. Wiers. 2011. Addiction, adolescence, and the integration of control and motivation. *Developmental Cognitive Neuroscience* 1:364–376.

Green, T. A., and S. Schenk. 2002. Dopaminergic mechanism for caffeine-produced cocaine seeking in rats. *Neuropsychopharmacology* 26(4):422–430.

Griffiths, R. R., S. M. Evans, S. J. Heishman, K. L. Preston, C. A. Sannerud, B. Wolf, and P. P. Woodson. 1990. Low-dose caffeine physical dependence in humans. *Journal of Pharmacology and Experimental Therapeutics* 255:1123–1132.

Haskell, C. F., D. O. Kennedy, A. L. Milne, K. A. Wesnes, and A. B. Scholey. 2008. The effects of L-theanine, caffeine and their combination on cognition and mood. *Biological Psychology* 77(2):113–122.

Hughes, J. R., A. H. Oliveto, A. Liguori, J. Carpenter, and T. Howard. 1998. Endorsement of DMS-IV dependence criteria among caffeine users. *Drug and Alcohol Dependence* 52:99–107.

Johnson, S. B., R. W. Blum, and J. N. Giedd. 2009. Adolescent maturity and the brain: The promise and pitfalls of neuroscience research in adolescent health policy. *Journal of Adolescent Health* 45:216–221.

Jones, H. A., and C. W. Lejuez. 2005. Personality correlates of caffeine dependence: The role of sensation seeking, impulsivity, and risk taking. *Experimental and Clinical Psychopharmacology* 13:259–266.

Jones, H. E., and R. R. Griffiths. 2003. Oral caffeine maintenance potentiates the reinforcing and stimulant subjective effects of intravenous nicotine in cigarette smokers. *Psychopharmacology* 165(3):280–290.

Juliano, L. M., and R. R. Griffiths. 2004. A critical review of caffeine withdrawal: Empirical validation of symptoms and signs, incidence, severity, and associated features. *Psychopharmacology* 176:1–29.

Juliano, L. M., D. P. Evatt, B. D. Richards, and R. R. Griffiths. 2012. Characterization of individuals seeking treatment for caffeine dependence. *Psychology of Addictive Behaviors* 26:948–954.

Karcz-Kubicha, M., K. Antoniou, A. Terasmaa, D. Quarta, M. Solinas, Z. Justinova, A. Pezzola, R. Reggio, C. E. Müller, K. Fuxe, S. R. Goldberg, P. Popoli, and S. Ferré. 2003. Involvement of adenosine A1 and A2A receptors in the motor effects of caffeine after its acute and chronic administration. *Neuropsychopharmacology* 28:1281–1291.

Kuhn, D. 2006. Do cognitive changes accompany developments in the adolescent brain? *Perspectives on Psychological Science* 1:59–67.

Lieberman, H. R., W. J. Tharion, B. Shukitt-Hale, K. L. Speckman, and R. Tulley. 2002. Effects of caffeine, sleep loss, and stress on cognitive performance and mood during U.S. Navy Seal training. *Psychopharmacology* 164:250–261.

Meredith, S. E., L. M. Juliano, J. R. Hughes, and R. R. Griffiths. 2013. Caffeine use disorder: A comprehensive review and research agenda. *Journal of Caffeine Research* 3(3):114–130.

Miller, K. E. 2008. Wired: Energy drinks, jock identity, masculine norms, and risk taking. *Journal of American College Health* 56:481–489.

Navarro, G., S. Ferré, A. Cordomi, E. Moreno, J. Mallol, V. Casadó, A. Cortés, H. Hoffmann, J. Ortiz, E. I. Canela, C. Lluis, L. Pardo, R. Franco, and A. S. Woods. 2010. Interactions between intracellular domains as key determinants of the quaternary structure and function of receptor heteromers. *Journal of Biological Chemistry* 285:27346–27359.

Orrú, M., J. Bakešová, M. Brugarolas, C. Quiroz, V. Beaumont, S. R. Goldberg, C. Lluis, A. Cortés, R. Franco, V. Casadó, E. I. Canela, and S. Ferré. 2011. Striatal pre- and post-synaptic profile of adenosine A(2A) receptor antagonist. *PLoS ONE* 6:e16088.

Orrú, M., X. Guitart, M. Karcz-Kubicha, M. Solinas, Z. Justinova, S. K. Barodia, J. Zanoveli, A. Cortes, C. Lluis, V. Casado, F. G. Moeller, and S. Ferré. 2013. Psychostimulant pharmacological profile of paraxanthine, the main metabolite of caffeine in humans. *Neuropharmacology* 67:476–484.

Panek, L. M., C. Swoboda, A. Bendlin, and J. L. Temple. 2013. Caffeine increases liking and consumption of novel-flavored yogurt. *Psychopharmacology (Berl)* 227:425–436.

Peacock, A., R. Bruno, F. H. Martin, and A. Carr. 2013. The impact of alcohol and energy drink consumption on intoxication and risk-taking behavior. *Alcoholism: Clinical and Experimental Research* 37(7):1234-1242.

Pharo, H., C. Sim, M. Graham, J. Gross, and H. Hayne. 2011. Risky business: Executive function, personality, and reckless behavior during adolescence and emerging adulthood. *Behavioral Neuroscience* 125:970–978.

Rogers, P. J., S. V. Heatherley, E. L. Mullings, and J. E. Smith. 2013. Faster but not smarter: Effects of caffeine and caffeine withdrawal on alertness and performance. *Psychopharmacology* 226(2):229–240.

Sigmon, S. C., R. I. Herning, W. Better, J. L. Cadet, and R. R. Griffiths. 2009. Caffeine withdrawal, acute effects, tolerance, and absence of net beneficial effects of chronic administration: Cerebral blood flow velocity, quantitative EEG, and subjective effects. *Pharmacology* 204(4):573–585.

Silverman, K., S. M. Evans, E. C. Strain, and R. R. Griffiths. 1992. Withdrawal syndrome after the double-blind cessation of caffeine consumption. *New England Journal of Medicine* 327:1109–1114.

Smit, H. J., and P. J. Rogers. 2000. Effects of low doses of caffeine on cognitive performance, mood and thirst in low and higher caffeine consumers. *Psychopharmacology* 152(2):167–173.

Smith, A. P. 2005. Caffeine at work. *Human Psychopharmacology* 20:441–445.

Smith, A. P., P. Brockman, R. Flynn, A. Maben, and M. Thomas. 1993. An investigation of the effects of coffee on alertness and performance during the day and night. *Neuropsychobiology* 27:217–233.

Solinas, M., S. Ferré, Z. B. You, M. Karcz-Kubicha, P. Popoli, and S. R. Goldberg. 2002. Caffeine induces dopamine and glutamate release in the shell of the nucleus accumbens. *Journal of Neuroscience* 22:6321–6324.

Spear, L. P. 2013. Adolescent neurodevelopment. *Journal of Adolescent Health* 52:s7–s13.

Stasio, M. J., K. I. M. Curr, A. L. Wagener, and D. M. Glassman. 2011. Revving up and staying up: Energy drink use associated with anxiety and sleep quality in a college sample. *College Student Journal* 45(4):738–748.

Steinberg, L. 2008. A social neuroscience perspective on adolescent risk-taking. *Developmental Review* 28:78–106.

Strain, E. C., G. K. Mumford, K. Silverman, and R. R. Griffiths. 1994. Caffeine dependence syndrome: Evidence from case histories and experimental evaluations. *Journal of the American Medical Association* 272:1043–1048.

Striley, C. L. W., R. R. Griffiths, and L. B. Cottler. 2011. Evaluating dependence criteria for caffeine. *Journal of Caffeine Research* 1:219–225.

Sturman, D. A., and B. Moghaddam. 2011. The neurobiology of adolescence: Changes in brain architecture, functional dynamics, and behavioral tendencies. *Neuroscience and Biobehavioral Reviews* 35:1704–1712.

Svikis, D. S., N. Berger, N. A. Haug, and R. R. Griffiths. 2005. Caffeine dependence in combination with a family history of alcoholism as a predictor of continued use of caffeine during pregnancy. *American Journal of Psychiatry* 162:2344–2351.

Temple, J. L., A. M. Bulkley, L. Briatico, and A. M. Dewey. 2009. Sex differences in reinforcing value of caffeinated beverages in adolescents. *Behavioural Pharmacology* 20:731–741.

Temple, J. L., A. M. Dewey, and L. N. Briatico. 2010. Effects of acute caffeine administration on adolescents. *Experimental and Clinical Psychopharmacology* 18:510–520.

Temple, J. L., A. M. Ziegler, A. Graczyk, A. Bendlin, S. O'Leary, and Y. S. Schnittker. 2012. Influence of caffeine on the liking of novel-flavored soda in adolescents. *Psychopharmacology (Berl)* 223:37–45.

Velazquez, C. E., N. S. Poulos, L. A. Latimer, and K. E. Pasch. 2012. Associations between energy drink consumption and alcohol use behaviors among college students. *Drug and Alcohol Dependence* 123(1–3):167–172.

Waring, W. S., J. Goudsmit, J. Marwick, D. J. Webb, and S. R. Maxwell. 2003. Acute caffeine intake influences central more than peripheral blood pressure in young adults. *American Journal of Hypertension* 16(11 Pt 1):919–924.

Wesensten, N., G. Blenky, M.A. Kautz, D.R. Thorne, R.M. Reichardt, and T. J. Balkin. 2002. Maintaining alertness and performance during sleep depreva-tion: Modafinil versus caffeine. *Psychopharmacology* 159(3):238–247.

White, A. M. 2009. Understanding adolescent brain development and its implications for the clinician. *Adolescent Medicine* 20:73–90.

Woods, A. S., and S. Ferré. 2005. Amazing stability of the arginine-phosphate electrostatic interaction. *Journal of Proteome Research* 4:1397–1402.

Woolsey, C. L., L. B. Barnes, B. H. Jacobson, W. S. Kensinger, A. E. Barry, N. C. Beck, A. G. Resnik, and M. W. Evans, Jr. 2013. Frequency of energy drink use predicts illicit prescription stimulant use. *Substance Abuse*, http://www.tandfonline.com/doi/abs/10.1080/08897077.2013.810561#preview (accessed December 22, 2013).

Yeomans, M. R. 2004. Understanding individual differences in acquired flavour liking in humans. *Appetite* 3(1):34–41.

Yeomans, M. R., A. Jackson, M. D. Lee, B. Steer, E. Tinley, P. Durlach, and P. J. Rogers. 2000. Acquisition and extinction of flavour preferences conditioned by caffeine in humans. *Appetite* 35(2):131–141.

Yeomans, M. R., T. Ripley, M. D. Lee, and P. J. Durlach. 2001. No evidence for latent learning of liking for flavours conditioned by caffeine. *Psychopharmacology* 157(2):172–179.

7

Other Compounds Impacting Caffeine Effects

Caffeinated food and beverage products on the market contain multiple compounds, with different products containing different types of compounds, which can have implications for the range and severity of health effects related to exposure. In the Day 2, Session 1, panel, moderated by Stephen Schaffer, Ph.D., University of South Alabama, Mobile, panelists considered whether and how those other compounds impact the health effects of caffeine on behavior and physiology. This chapter summarizes Schaffer's opening remarks, the panelists' remarks, and the discussion that followed. Although all caffeinated foods and beverages contain other ingredients, the focus of the session was on caffeine-containing energy drinks and other products with added sources of caffeine. Box 7-1 reviews key points made by speakers.

INTERACTION BETWEEN ENERGY DRINK INGREDIENTS AND CAFFEINE

Presented by Stephen Schaffer, Ph.D.,
University of South Alabama

Several times throughout the workshop, participants considered whether the health effects of caffeine-containing energy drinks and other products with added caffeine are different from those of coffee and other products with naturally existing caffeine. Answering that question requires, first, knowing what the ingredients are. Stephen Schaffer provided an overview of common ingredients in caffeine-containing energy

BOX 7-1
Key Points Made by Individual Speakers

- In Stephen Schaffer's opinion, evidence reported in the scientific literature suggests that most other ingredients in caffeinated energy drinks (i.e., ingredients besides caffeine) appear to inhibit the potential adverse effects of caffeine. Clinical studies are rare, however.
- Carl Keen emphasized the "moving target" nature of caffeinated energy drink ingredients as a result of competitive marketing. He also reminded the workshop audience of the complex mixtures of ingredients in coffee, tea, cocoa, and other products with naturally existing caffeine. The food industry is constantly changing not just the ingredients being used in those other types of products but also the way those products are processed. He warned against extrapolating results from studies of caffeine (or any other ingredient) conducted in one product to other products.
- John Higgins emphasized that results from in vivo studies often differ from in vitro study results. He echoed other calls for more clinical studies.
- While clinical studies on the effects of combinations of caffeine and other ingredients are rare, they are even rarer in the context of pregnancy. Christina Chambers called for more research in pregnant populations. Although it is unethical to conduct randomized clinical trials among pregnant women, she said, "We can do a much better job of conducting observational studies."
- Given the lack of data on whether and how caffeinated energy drink ingredients are associated with cardiac death, for Jeffrey Goldberger the question is: how can those data be collected? He called for a clinical assessment to determine whether the reported observations of cardiac death create a signal suggesting that there might be an association. Then, if an association exists, is it causal? What are the potential mechanisms? Given the likely rare risk of cardiac death, a surrogate risk biomarker (i.e., a biomarker associated with the end point of interest) would be a useful tool for conducting clinical studies.

drinks and what is known—and not known—about those ingredients and their interactions with caffeine. He focused on glucuronolactone, taurine, vitamins, and herbal extracts (e.g., ginseng, guarana, and ginko biloba). In sum, he concluded that, in his view, these other ingredients inhibit some of the potential adverse effects of caffeine. But clinical studies are rare, he said, and more are needed.

Glucuronolactone

There is not much known about glucuronolactone, according to Schaffer. It was initially added to energy drinks to improve mood and diminish fatigue. Glucuronolactone is a naturally occurring substance and is a major component of connective tissue. Derived from glucose, glucuronolactone is metabolized in humans via the pentose pathway, with some of the products of that pathway, xylitol in particular, having important physiological effects. Xylitol is a pancreatic secretagogue of insulin. In rodents, but not in humans, xylitol is converted into ascorbic acid.

Normally, humans are exposed to about 38 mg per day, with average energy drink consumers exposed to about 126 mg per day. Among heavy energy drink consumers, that is, those in the 95th percentile, exposure is quite high, about 840 to 900 mg per day. With respect to toxicity, according to Schaffer there has been only one real study, a 13-week oral toxicity study in rats conducted in Europe by the Scientific Committee on Food. The researchers found that, at higher doses, vacuoles formed in the kidneys. In a follow-up study, the researchers did not detect any vacuolization but did observe some focal inflammation of the kidney. On the basis of those results, the committee concluded that exposure below 300 mg per kg of body mass is completely safe. Schaffer observed that levels of glucuronolactone in energy drinks are well below that level. He was not aware of any studies examining the interaction between glucuronolactone and caffeine.

Taurine

Schaffer described taurine as a "very simple compound" formed from cysteine via decarboxylation and oxidation of the sulfhydryl group. Taurine has several physiological functions: bile acid conjugation, osmoregulation (with tremendous amounts of taurine present in the heart and brain, as high as 10 millimolar concentrations, but micromolar concentrations in plasma), neural modulation, inflammation, and mitochondrial function. Schaffer emphasized the important role that taurine serves in the mitochondria, where it conjugates with uridines at the wobble position on tRNA and thereby enhances codon-anticodon interactions and synthesis of respiratory chain proteins. Taurine deficiency leads to poor respiratory chain flux, which in turn leads to decreased oxygen consumption and decreased adenosine triphosphate synthesis. In addition, electrons are diverted from the respiratory chain to oxygen, resulting in the formation of super oxide and the creation of oxidated stress. Ultimately, taurine deficiency is associated with a number of pathological conditions: retinopathy, cardiomyopathy, myopathy, immune deficiency, and development defects.

Furthermore, noted Schaffer, children, adolescents, and adults eating omnivorous diets consume anywhere from 40 to 400 mg of taurine per day. Average energy drink consumers are exposed to about 270–280 mg daily, and heavy energy drink consumers (i.e., in the 95th percentile) are exposed to 1,400–2,300 mg daily.

Schaffer described the elimination of taurine, which is dose dependent. If administered 30 mg per kg of body mass within the first 6 hours, 20 to 30 percent is eliminated in the urine; if administered 300 mg per kg body mass, 40 to 50 percent is eliminated in the urine (Sved et al., 2007). Only a small amount of ingested taurine enters tissues. Even after 14 days of 300 mg per day exposure, the levels of taurine in the brain and heart remain constant (Sved et al., 2007). In 2009, the European Food Safety Authority (EFSA) stated that taurine (3–6 g) had been administered daily to a large group of patients, including adults, children, and even infants, with no noted no adverse health effects (EFSA, 2009).

With respect to potential interactions between taurine and caffeine, probably the best studied, in Schaffer's opinion, is diuresis and natriuresis. Taurine was demonstrated to be a weak diuretic and natriuretic by Mozaffari and Schaffer (2001), in a comparison of fluid and sodium excretion rates between taurine-depleted and taurine-supplemented animals. Nonetheless, he also opined that Mozaffari and Schaffer (2001) tested taurine levels that one would not ordinarily see among individuals consuming energy drinks. With respect to the diuretic potential of a taurine-caffeine combination, Schaffer identified Riesenhuber et al. (2006) as an especially well-designed clinical study and encouraged more such studies. The researchers administered energy drinks to study participants, with some energy drinks lacking caffeine, some lacking taurine, and some lacking both. They found that taurine did not significantly impact urine output or natruresis.

According to Schaffer, there has been concern expressed in the literature about the potential effects of taurine on blood pressure and heart rate. Using taurine-deficient rats, Mozaffari et al. (2006) showed that taurine deficiency leads to increased blood pressure. In humans, Yamori et al. (2010) showed that increased taurine excretion led to decreased blood pressure among individuals with higher blood pressure but that increased taurine excretion had no impact on blood pressure in individuals with normal heart rates. In addition, studies with spontaneous hypertensive animals have demonstrated that the addition of taurine leads to decreased blood pressure. With respect to the combined effect of taurine and caffeine on blood pressure and heart rate, Bichler et al. (2006) demonstrated decreased heart rate without a change in blood pressure when taurine and caffeine were administered in combination. Nevertheless, according to Schaffer, it is difficult to extract a lot of information from the study because the researchers did not examine taurine and caffeine individually, only in combination.

Schaffer pointed out that cardiac arrhythmias are another potential effect of concern. Although the ingestion of caffeine is a common cause of ectopic heart beats, arrhythmias are also produced by nutrient deficiencies, including taurine deficiency (Eby and Halcomb, 2006).

Basal spasms, he said, have been identified in the literature as yet another potential problem. Calcium antagonists are one way to treat basal spasms. Abebe (2008) demonstrated in rats that taurine does not affect aortic tension, regardless of whether calcium is present, except in the case of diabetes. In rats with diabetes, taurine actually reduced vascular tension.

Finally, some researchers have expressed concern that taurine-caffeine interactions may affect seizures. L'Amoreaux et al. (2010) found that taurine prolonged latency to seizure when both injected subcutaneously (43 mg per kg) and fed to animals (water containing 0.05 percent taurine). According to Schaffer, that is good range of exposure levels. The researchers found that the effect was related to chlorine transports, with taurine actually interacting or competing with picrotoxin at the GABA receptor. El Idrissi et al. (2003) had previously found that chronic feeding of taurine led to an increase in GABA. Schaffer explained that either GABA itself acts as an inhibitor, thereby decreasing seizures, or, as El Idrissi et al. (2003) suggested, the GABA receptor is down-regulated.

Herbal Supplements

Schaffer described herbal supplements in caffeinated energy drinks, including guarana, the seeds of which contain greater amounts of caffeine than coffee beans do (Woods, 2012). When added to energy drinks, guarana increases the amount of metabolized caffeine.

Another herbal supplement, ginseng, contains a number of steroids, one of which is ginsenoside-Rg1, which can bind to the glucocorticoid receptor and displace dexamethasone (Lee et al., 1997). At the right concentration, ginseng may have an anti-inflammatory effect. Hong et al. (2012) demonstrated a concentration-dependent reduction in blood pressure, but at doses too high to be relevant. Lian et al. (2005) demonstrated a concentration-dependent increased latency to seizures.

Finally, Schaffer sought evidence for the effects of ginkgo biloba. He did not find much. Krieglstein et al. (1986) reported increased cerebral blood flow in rats, and Braquet (1993) reported inhibited platelet activation. But again, the effects were at concentrations too high to be relevant, according to Schaffer.

PANELIST REMARKS

Carl L. Keen, Ph.D.,
University of California, Davis

Carl Keen stressed the importance of the fact that, although Schaffer covered some of the major compounds of today's energy drinks, "this will be a very moveable target." Because of market competition, energy drinks on the market 6 months or 1 year from now may have very different compositions. Already he has seen energy drinks with ingredients such as beet root and pomegranate juice, added for their vasodilation effects. He cautioned against pigeonholing energy drinks with respect to other compounds that may or may not interact with caffeine.

Keen also called attention to the fact that energy drinks are not the only caffeinated food or dietary supplement. Coffee, tea, and cocoa are just three examples of the many others. All of those are complex mixtures with thousands of compounds, many of which can have synergistic, neutral, or antagonistic effects with caffeine. For example, some of the catechins and the theobromine present in coffee, tea, and cocoa have very potent vascular effects that typically increase endothelial relaxation. Those potential effects are important to keep in mind when evaluating the epidemiological literature, in Keen's opinion. Studies that report only on coffee consumption, for example, ignore the fact that the processing of that coffee, as well as the temperature at which it is served, can change the profile of some of the other compounds, particularly the catechins. The catechins could end up having either very strong endothelial relaxation properties or zero endothelial relaxation properties. Plus, the food industry is always trying to develop new methodologies that might alter the profiles of some of these compounds. In Keen's opinion, not only do these new methodologies have implications for how older epidemiology studies are interpreted, but they also have implications for how future controlled intervention studies are designed.

Keen echoed other workshop participant cautionary calls that extrapolating results from studies on caffeine in isolation to caffeine in food products is, as he said, "fraught with error." Indeed, it is opposite to what a recent Institute of Medicine study on biomarkers recommended, that is, when evaluating compounds, whether it be caffeine or something else, it should be done within the framework of the food being evaluated (IOM, 2010).

John P. Higgins, M.D., M.B.A.

University of Texas Medical School, Houston

John Higgins reiterated what Schaffer had stated about the lack of clinical studies on many of the other compounds present in caffeine-containing energy drinks. A lesson learned in cardiology is that findings from in vitro studies do not always hold true in clinical trials. Effects are often very different in the human system than in a test tube. Moreover, not only is the human system different from a test tube, but human system dynamics vary among individuals in numerous ways; variables include, for example, genetically, by age, sex, exposure (e.g., exposure to pure caffeine versus coffee versus energy beverage), and other toxicities that the body may also be dealing with at the time.

As an example of different results obtained in vitro versus in vivo, Higgins mentioned a study of 9 individuals who consumed either an energy drink with 80 mg of caffeine and 1,000 mg of taurine or a control containing 80 mg pure caffeine (Franks et al., 2012). The researchers reported that blood pressure was significantly greater among individuals who consumed the energy drink versus pure caffeine. In another study, researchers compared the cardiovascular effects during exercise of the energy drink with taurine to the effects of another similar energy beverage but without any taurine (Baum and Weiss, 2001). They reported a significant increase in contractility and a higher stroke volume in the group that had the energy drink with taurine, which meant, as Higgins explained, that the heart had to work harder, that is, cardiac work (and its maximal oxygen consumption) is proportional to contractility, so greater contractility means greater work for the heart. Finally, Higgins mentioned a case report of a 28-year-old motocross cycle rider in Australia who was drinking energy beverages throughout the day and experienced a ventricular cardiac arrest (Berger and Alford, 2009). Tests conducted in the hospital indicated that he had experienced some kind of abnormal vascular functioning. It was postulated that the combination of exercise and the consumption of a caffeine- and taurine-containing beverage had interacted and led to a heart attack.

Higgins encouraged more human studies on the interactions between caffeine and other compounds. Such studies may also help researchers understand why some individuals are more vulnerable to various types of caffeine exposures.

Christina Chambers, Ph.D., M.P.H.

University of California, San Diego

Building on what Keen and Higgins said, Christina Chambers remarked that, in the context of pregnancy, "I can sum it up by saying there's almost no data." The lack of data during pregnancy is typical for most prescription medicines, let alone for herbal and other products, despite that an estimated one-quarter to one-third of all pregnant women consume some type of herbal product. It makes it difficult to say anything about the safety, or lack of safety, during human pregnancy of any of these compounds either by themselves or in combination with caffeine. Compounding the challenge, Chambers noted, is what Keen had said about the moving-target nature of the research, and she remarked that the (caffeinated energy drink) products are "changing probably as we speak."

Chambers called for more human data on the effects of such products as energy drinks that contain multiple compounds. Although it would be unethical to conduct randomized clinical trials in the pregnant population, she said, "We can do a much better job of conducting observational studies."

Chambers also raised an additional issue: the consumption of energy drinks in combination with alcohol. She observed that the use of energy drinks in combination with alcohol appears to attenuate the depressant effects of alcohol, with one recent study reporting that adults who consume energy drinks in combination with alcohol are more likely to binge drink. Given that more than half of all pregnancies in the United States are unplanned, the potential for a woman to drink like that, that is, to consume alcohol in combination with an energy drink, raises some concern.

Jeffrey Goldberger, M.D.
Northwestern University, Chicago, Illinois

Jeffrey Goldberger reiterated what he had said earlier during his presentation about the lack of data suggesting an elevated risk of cardiac arrhythmia following the consumption of an energy beverage, but he framed his claim differently. He explained what he referred to as the statistical basis for that statement. That is, studies are conducted that compare the number of events that occur in people who are exposed to a substance versus people who are not exposed to that substance, and odds ratios are calculated that indicate whether the people exposed have an increased, decreased, or no difference in risk. The important thing to keep in mind is that, regardless of the calculated odds ratio, researchers also calculate what is known as a 95 percent confidence interval, that is, a range of odds ratio values within which one can be 95 percent sure that the true odds ratio is somewhere in that interval. For example, if a study shows absolutely no difference in risk of sudden cardiac death between those exposed to coffee and those not exposed to coffee, then the odds ratio would be 1. Suppose further that the researchers calculated a very tight 95 percent confidence interval: 0.99–1.01. That means that, according to the data, one can be 95 percent sure that the true odds ratio is between 0.99 and 1.01. But one cannot be 100 percent sure.

Goldberger observed that, at this point, it remains a huge question whether any caffeinated energy beverages are associated with an increased risk of sudden cardiac death. If an increased risk exists, in Goldberger's opinion, it is "probably very small." Otherwise, given how much exposure there has been to caffeinated energy beverages, it would already be detectable. "If one is concerned about the small potential increase in risk related to sudden cardiac death," he said, "one has to come up with a strategy that would be able to address that very, very small increased risk."

He stressed the importance of collecting observations, such as the case report mentioned by Higgins, and then conducting clinical assessments to evaluate those observations and determine whether together they create a signal to suggest that there might be an association. Then, if there is an association, is it causal? Goldberger encouraged the identification of surrogate markers for risk, given that surrogate markers associated with end points of interest are especially helpful for very rare events. As an example, he pointed to the association between liquid protein diets and sudden cardiac death and how researchers discovered that liquid protein diets cause QT prolongation and that QT prolongation was identified as a marker for the risk of sudden cardiac death.

PANELIST DISCUSSION WITH THE AUDIENCE

Following the panelists' remarks, audience members were invited to ask questions of the panelists. Topics covered ranged from the challenge of detecting a small health risk (i.e., sudden cardiac death) to the "demonizing" of energy drinks and the need for an assessment of the science of the safety of caffeine exposure to consider all of the many different types of food and beverages that contain caffeine.

The Challenge of Detecting a Small Health Risk

A member of the audience commented on the large number of energy drinks being sold compared to the very small number of sudden cardiac deaths being reported. He said, "I'm concerned about trying to match the magnitude of a phenomenon as large as the number sold against minor anecdotes and basic research that is not related to what's happening in the clinical arena." According to the commenter, there are 350,000 sudden cardiac deaths annually. Among those, he said, "you could find somebody who had an energy drink that day." In his opinion, "there's no disease." Another audience member questioned why, with 50 billion energy drinks being sold worldwide and 20 million being sold in the United States, no clusters [of effects] are being seen, for example, on college campuses.

In response, Goldberger reiterated that if there is a risk, it is a small risk. The lack of an apparent large signal does not rule out the possibility of, in Goldberger's words, a "very, very small effect." He speculated that data related to coffee consumption in adult populations, which he identified as the largest collection of data (related to the health effects of caffeine exposure), are probably consistent with a one-tenth of 1 percent increased risk in sudden cardiac death (but has not been demonstrated). That same risk (if real) would probably also exist in relation to other forms of caffeine. The challenge to detecting the possibility of low-level risks is lack of data. He considered it "reasonable" to begin to track events associated with different forms of caffeine and continue to collect information and then decide whether the formulations are different.

There were several calls for a registry to track adverse effects associated with the consumption of energy drinks and other caffeine-containing foods and beverages. For example, Steven Lipshultz suggested that sudden cardiac death be tracked via postmarketing surveillance.

Effects of Taurine on Cardiac End Points: The Need for More Research

Higgins was asked about his interpretation of Baum and Weiss (2001), that is, that an increase in stroke volume was more work for the heart. The commenter's understanding was that an increased stroke volume for the same amount of work would actually lead to a decrease in the afterload and would, thus, be beneficial. Higgins explained that stroke volume, heart rate, and blood pressure all increased in the group who consumed the energy drink with taurine and that those individuals were doing more work for the same amount of exercise. Myocardial oxygen consumption is determined by maximal heart rate and blood pressure (or rate pressure product). Thus, the energy drink with taurine resulted in higher cardiac work, higher oxygen consumption, for the same amount of exercise done by both groups. He concluded that this was excess or unnecessary work in the group who had the energy drink with taurine. He compared it to "flogging a dead horse." Consumption of the energy drink appeared to be causing excessive stimulation, more than was needed for the amount of exercise being done. When asked whether an increased stroke volume would be advantageous for someone participating in a bike time trial or very competitive race, Higgins replied that more studies would need to be done to answer that question.

Schaffer commented on the fact that, according to Higgins, the only difference between the two treatment groups was taurine (i.e., individuals who consumed the energy drink with taurine were exposed to taurine, whereas individuals who consumed pure caffeine were not). According to Schaffer, taurine enhances mitochondrial function, which means it enhances respiratory chain function. During exercise, the heart is somewhat hypoxic. If what oxygen is available could be used in a better way to produce adenosine triphosphate, the heart would benefit. Again, Higgins said that he could not comment because, as far as he was aware, the researchers did not measure that actual effect.

Are the Concentrations of Other Ingredients in Energy Drinks Great Enough to Have Physiological Effects?

A member of the audience asked whether some of the other ingredients in caffeinated energy drinks, such as taurine, are added primarily as a way to include their name on the label and give consumers the impression that there is something special about a product. Are their concentrations great enough to affect taste or to have physiological effects? He also questioned whether it is legal to add ingredients that are being added for their druglike effects. Schaffer replied that, for ginseng, extracts contain different mixes of steroids depending on how the ginseng is extracted. In the study he mentioned on ginseng and seizures (Lian et al., 2005), the researchers administered 20 mg of extract per kg, which he said is within the range of what is added to energy drinks. He did not know which type of ginseng extract is used in energy drinks.

What About Sugar?

An audience member commented on the reinforcing properties of caffeine, with young males reporting that they preferred sodas with greater caffeine content and with what she referred to as sugar's "natural reward system." She suggested that the interaction between caffeine and sugar could have important implications for obesity and diabetes, with caffeine reinforcing the natural reward system of sugar. Higgins mentioned that the topic has been covered in the literature. He noted that sugar contents vary among different concoctions. For example, sports drinks often have 6 to 8 percent carbohydrate concentration, which appears to be optimal for absorption during exercise, and energy drinks tend to have about 11 to 12 percent. He mentioned one study showing that the ergogenic benefits of caffeine during exercise appear to be reduced when combined with carbohydrates, although they may improve in exercise of longer duration. Another study showed that caffeine absorption into circulation may be slowed and removal from circulation accelerated when caffeine is consumed with large amounts of glucose. So, there does appear to be some interaction between caffeine and glucose.

The Value of In Vitro Versus In Vivo Studies

In response to the several calls for more clinical studies, an audience member emphasized that in vivo studies would not be possible without in vitro studies. The same is true of preclinical animal studies. Phase I clinical trials are safety studies that can only be conducted after preclinical animal data have been collected.

Higgins replied that most two-compound studies have been conducted only in vitro—for example, studies on the effects of combining caffeine and taurine—and it is likely that there may be other interactions in vivo that may result in different effects.

Goldberger pointed to sudden cardiac death as a very complex condition affected by multiple factors. Even though long QT syndrome is a risk factor for sudden cardiac death, a person can live with long QT syndrome for years until suddenly, seemingly out of nowhere, sudden cardiac death appears. Many factors must converge at a particular time in order to create that environment. Even if sudden cardiac death is related to caffeine ingestion, it probably emerges in people who have been ingesting caffeine for years. The complexity of the problem and the challenge of ferreting out these factors need to be part of the analysis and consideration.

Criticism of Energy Drinks

An audience member commented on the "cherry picking" of references that is sometimes done to make a point and the "demonizing" of certain groups of products, namely, energy drinks. That approach is not helpful. There are many different types of caffeinated foods and beverages, and an assessment of the science of the safety of caffeine exposure should consider all these different sources.

REFERENCES

Abebe, W. 2008. Effects of taurine on the reactivity of aortas from diabetic rats. *Life Sciences* 82:279–289.

Baum, M., and M. Weiss. 2001. The influence of a taurine containing drink on cardiac parameters before and after exercise measured by echocardiography. *Amino Acids* 20(1):75–82.

Berger, A. J., and K. Alford. 2009. Cardiac arrest in a young man following excess consumption of caffeinated "energy drinks." *Medical Journal of Australia* 190:41–43.

Bichler, A., A. Swenson, and M. A. Harris. 2006. A combination of caffeine and taurine has no effect on short-term memory but induces changes in heart rate and mean arterial blood pressure. *Amino Acids* 31:471–476.

Braquet, P. 1993. Cedemin, a *Ginkgo biloba* extract, should not be considered as a PAF antagonist. *American Journal of Gastroenterology* 88:2138.

Eby, G., and W. W. Halcomb. 2006. Elimination of cardiac arrhythmias using oral taurine with l-arginine with case histories: Hypothesis for nitric oxide stabilization of the sinus node. *Medical Hypotheses* 67:1200–1204.

EFSA (European Food Safety Authority). 2009. The use of taurine and D-glucurono-gamma-lactone as constituents of the so-called "energy" drinks. *EFSA Journal* 935:1–31. http://www.efsa.europa.eu/en/scdocs/doc/935.pdf (accessed February 11, 2014).

El Idrissi, A., J. Messing, J. Scalia, and E. Trenkner. 2003. Prevention of epileptic seizures by taurine. *Advances in Experimental Medicine and Biology* 526:515–525.

Franks, A. M., J. M. Schmidt, K. R. McCain, and M. Fraer. 2012. Comparison of the effects of energy drink versus caffeine supplementation on indices of 24-hour ambulatory blood pressure. *Annals of Pharmacotherapy* 46:192–199.

Hong, S. Y., Y. Y. Kim, H. Y. Ahn, J. H. Shin, and O. Kwon. 2012. Panax ginseng extract rich in ginsenoside protopanaxatriol attenuates blood pressure elevation in spontaneously hypertensive rats by affecting the Akt-dependent phosphorylation of endothelial nitric oxide synthase. *Journal of Agricultural and Food Chemistry* 60:3086–3091.

IOM (Institute of Medicine). 2010. *Evaluation of biomarkers and surrogate endpoints in chronic disease.* Washington, DC: The National Academies Press.

Krieglstein, J., T. Beck, and A. Seibert. 1986. Influence of an extract of *Ginkgo biloba* on cerebral blood flow and metabolism. *Life Sciences* 39:2327–2334.

L'Amoreaux, W. J., A. Marsillo, and A. El Idrissi. 2010. Pharmacological characterization of GABAA receptors in taurine-fed mice. *Journal of Biomedical Science* 17(Supp 1):S14. doi: 10.1186/1423-0127-17-S1-S14. http://www.ncbi.nlm.nih.gov/pmc/articles/PMC2994404 (accessed February 11, 2014).

Lee, Y. J., E. Chung, K. Y. Lee, Y. H. Lee, B. Huh, and S. K. Lee. 1997. Ginsenoside-Rg1, one of the major active molecules from Panax ginseng, is a functional ligand of glucocorticoid receptor. *Molecular and Cellular Endocrinology* 133:135–140.

Lian, X. Y., Z. Z. Zhang, and J. L. Stringer. 2005. Anticonvulsant activity of ginseng on seizures induced by chemical convulsants. *Epilepsia* 46:15–22.

Mozaffari, M. S., and D. Schaffer. 2001. Taurine modulates arginine vasopressin-mediated regulation of renal function. *Journal of Cardiovascular Pharmacology* 37:742–750.

Mozaffari, M. S., C. Patel, R. Abdelsayed, and S. W. Schaffer. 2006. Accelerated NaCl-induced hypertension in taurine-deficient rat: Role of renal function. *Kidney International* 70:329–337.

Riesenhuber, A., M. Boehm, M. Posch, and C. Aufricht. 2006. Diuretic potential of energy drinks. *Amino Acids* 31:81–83.

Sved, D. W., J. L. Godsey, S. L. Ledyard, A. P. Mahoney, P. L. Stetson, S. Ho, N. R. Myers, P. Resnis, and A. G. Renwick. 2007. Absorption, tissue distribution, metabolism and elimination of taurine given orally to rats. *Amino Acids* 32:459–466.

Woods, D. J. 2012. Guarana: *Paullinia cupana, P. sorbilis*; also known as Brazilian cocoa and "zoom." *Journal of Primary Health Care* 4:163–164.

Yamori, Y., T. Taguchi, A. Hamada, K. Kunimasa, H. Mori, and M. Mori. 2010. Taurine in health and diseases: Consistent evidence from experimental and epidemiological studies. *Journal of Biomedical Science* 17 (Suppl 1):S6. doi:10.1186/1423-0127-17-S1-S6. http://www.ncbi.nlm.nih.gov/pmc/articles/PMC2994368 (accessed February 11, 2014).

8

Public Comments

At the end of Day 1, workshop participants were invited to comment on any issue, with 3 minutes provided per participant. This chapter summarizes comments made, in alphabetical order by the last name of the participant. Note that the observations and opinions expressed here are those of individual workshop participants.

RICHARD H. ADAMSON, Ph.D., TPN ASSOCIATES, LLC

Both roasted and brewed coffees have more than one thousand compounds, Richard Adamson reiterated. Caffeine is not even the most abundant compound in coffee. Chlorogenic acid, trigonelline, total peptides, and total carbohydrates are all present in greater quantities. Energy drinks, on the other hand, generally have only four or five ingredients, usually caffeine, taurine or another amino acid, glucose or another carbohydrate, sometimes glucuronolactone, and sometimes herbs. Caffeine is usually the only or central stimulant. There is very little evidence that any of those other ingredients have adverse effects. Adamson noted that both taurine and glucuronolactone have been examined several times by the European Food Safety Authority, which has established a no observed adverse effect level (NOAEL) of 1,000 mg per kg in animals and a safe level in humans of 100 mg per kg.

BOB ARNOT, M.D., MEDICAL ADVISOR TO MONSTER BEVERAGE, INC.

Bob Arnot found it particularly striking how little caffeine is consumed by adolescents and children. He clarified that the U.S. Food and Drug Administration (FDA) itself has recognized that several deaths recorded in the FDA Adverse Event Reporting System are not necessarily causally associated with caffeinated energy drinks. One of the two lawsuits launched against Monster Energy involves a 14-year-old girl who had myocarditis. Arnot said it is important to note that no link has been found between caffeine or other stimulants and myocarditis. The second case is a 19-year-old boy who had cardiomyopathy. The boy's lawyer alleged a causal effect resulting from 3 years of drinking energy drinks and consuming about 320 mg of caffeine per day. Again, in Arnot's opinion, there is no link between caffeine or caffeinated energy drinks and cardiomyopathy. The boy had other risk factors for cardiomyopathy.

JOEL GEERLING, M.D., Ph.D., HARVARD MEDICAL SCHOOL, BOSTON

Joel Geerling remarked that he had been following for a number of years the controversies in the literature regarding caffeinated energy drinks, partly because his colleagues and patients have questions about it and partly because he himself consumes caffeinated energy drinks. He switched from coffee to caffeinated energy drinks a number of years ago because of personal preference and because he likes the moderate and consistent amount of caffeine in energy drink cans compared to coffee purchased from a coffee shop. He expressed disappointment with much of what he has read in the literature, even in what he considers good peer-reviewed clinical journals. He has seen what he considers exaggerations and, in some cases, misstatements that have passed peer review. As an example, he mentioned an article published in *Pediatrics* a couple of years ago in which the authors stated that some children are at increased risk for cardiac arrhythmias and sudden death from caffeine-containing products (Seifert et al., 2011). According to Geerling, the authors cited three articles that did not even contain the word "caffeine," which Geerling found worrisome. He urged workshop participants to consider the content and quality of the evidence being discussed. One of the articles was about prenatal exposure to cocaine (Frassica et al.,

1994), and the other was about the ethics of treating children with cardiomyopathies (Lipshultz, 2000). He noticed that during the workshop discussion of behavioral survey data, no one mentioned what Geerling identified as the largest randomized controlled trial of caffeine administration to infants and children. The trial included behavioral outcomes. Geerling also referred to the many other randomized controlled trials conducted with intravenous caffeine that have found no causal association between caffeine and seizures.

JOHN P. HIGGINS, M.D., M.B.A., UNIVERSITY OF TEXAS MEDICAL SCHOOL, HOUSTON

John Higgins observed that the physician code of ethics includes "First, do no harm." He reiterated that caffeinated energy drinks are different from coffee. If coffee was dangerous, more issues would have emerged by now. Likewise with pure caffeine—it has a different effect. If physicians are to, first, do no harm, in Higgins's opinion, one of the first questions that needs to be asked is: Who is vulnerable? Even if just a small percentage of children and adolescents are vulnerable, for whatever reason, then why not consider doing what others have done and protect, as a society, that small percentage? Some countries have banned such drinks altogether, and others have banned their sale to individuals under the age of 18. Also, his understanding was that the 14-year-old girl involved in one of the two lawsuits against Monster Energy was diagnosed with Ehlers-Danlos syndrome, not myocarditis.

RICHARD KINGSTON, Pharm.D., SAFETYCALL INTERNATIONAL, BLOOMINGTON, MINNESOTA

Richard Kingston expressed concern that the poison control adverse event data presented by Alvin Bronstein (see Chapter 3 for a summary of Bronstein's presentation) excluded what Kingston considered two of the most important outcome categories: (1) nontoxic, no follow-up, asymptomatic outcomes, and (2) minor effect, no follow-up outcomes. The analysis presented by Bronstein was published in *Clinical Toxicology* (Bronstein et al., 2011), where all 1,480 nonalcoholic energy drink exposures are categorized into outcomes by age group.

According to Kingston, if the excluded outcomes are included, children less than 6 years of age had the lowest incidence of adverse effects even though they had the highest exposure rate. In fact, according to Kingston, 85 percent of cases involving children less than 6 years of age were either nontoxic or resulted in minor adverse consequences. When including the 6- to 12-year-old population, still greater than 80 percent of cases were nontoxic, and serious outcomes were rare. Leaving out these two outcome groups distorts the denominator and exaggerates the overall relative percentage of adverse effects in all populations, Kingston explained.

In his opinion, a more meaningful statistic would be to highlight the average age of all symptomatic exposure, which would likely demonstrate that older teenagers and adults should be the target populations for risk mitigation efforts. For the 13- to 20-year-old population, overall numbers of incidents were extremely low considering the ubiquitous availability of products. Even for the 249 cases tabulated, serious outcomes appear to be uncommon. In fact, for all populations, serious outcomes appear to be uncommon. In Kingston's opinion, seven major effects is small. He found the analysis further disappointing in that seven cases contained virtually no incident details, such as an indication of which products may have been involved, formulation characteristics, doses of caffeine, and other factors potentially contributing to the reported adverse effects.

In Kingston's opinion, a positive and important message from Bronstein's presentation is that more focused postmarket surveillance is needed to define which products and formulations give rise to adverse effects, especially in those populations routinely consuming such products. More focused postmarket surveillance would help to direct injury prevention methods to the appropriate populations.

EMILIA C. LONARDO, Ph.D., GROCERY MANUFACTURERS ASSOCIATION, WASHINGTON, DC

Caffeine has been part of the human diet for centuries, Emilia Lonardo remarked. It is a safe, naturally occurring substance found in leaves, seeds, or fruits of more than 60 plants, many of which are staples in the human diet. In addition to its natural presence in commonly consumed foods, caffeine is used as a food ingredient. Caffeine safety has been extensively studied, with more than 140 regulatory agencies worldwide considering the appropriate use of caffeine in food to be safe. Lonardo expressed the Grocery Manufacturers Association's willingness to work with the FDA on enhancing label information on caffeinated products so that consumers are more aware of the caffeine content in the products they enjoy and to collaborate with the FDA on developing a guidance document that sets appropriate boundaries for the addition of caffeine to food products. Such boundaries should be based on sound scientific evidence and in the best interest of public health.

REND AL-MONDHIRY, J.D., COUNCIL FOR RESPONSIBLE NUTRITION, WASHINGTON, DC

The Council for Responsible Nutrition (CRN) encourages balanced robust discussions on caffeine, continued research on caffeine in all sources and its potential effect on vulnerable populations, and examination of data gaps. Future policies and regulation should be based on sound science. The CRN believes that safety is paramount and, as such, supports the current regulatory framework, which helps to promote safe dietary supplement products, including those containing caffeine.

The CRN also recognizes the role of industry in ensuring safe products and the importance of transparency so that consumers, particularly parents, can make good decisions. At the manufacturing level, good manufacturing practices help to ensure high-quality products. Manufacturers are also required by law to ensure that products are safe before they are sold and that products are labeled appropriately. Al-Mondhiry noted that the CRN-recommended labeling guidelines for caffeine-containing dietary supplements play an important role in informing consumers, particularly parents, about the amount of caffeine in a particular supplement and alerting those who are sensitive to caffeine about the presence of caffeine in a product.

Finally, the CRN also supports mandatory adverse event reporting, which the council views as an effective and important way to monitor safety postmarket.

In closing, Al-Mondhiry expressed CRN's support of the type of dialogue being fostered at this workshop and looks forward to working with the FDA on any future guidance documents for these products.

J. PHILIP SAUL, M.D., UNIVERSITY OF SOUTH CAROLINA, MOUNT PLEASANT, AND CONSULTANT TO THE AMERICAN BEVERAGE ASSOCIATION

As a pediatric cardiologist, Phil Saul divides his patients into three groups: (1) patients under the age of 12, for whom he does not recommend caffeine but does not restrict chocolate; (2) patients between the ages of 12 and 18, for whom he recommends no caffeine only if the patient has an underlying cardiac condition (the three main conditions of concern being arrhythmias, syncope, and any kind of significant cardiomyopathy); and (3) other patients. Although evidence suggests that most arrhythmias are not exacerbated by caffeine, some are, and almost all physicians recommend that patients with arrhythmias avoid caffeinated beverages. Saul recommends slow withdrawal for patients with benign syncope, which is often exacerbated by caffeine.

Saul usually queries his patients about the types of beverages they consume because most patients between the age of 12 and 18 are not aware of caffeine in the products they are consuming. He observed that energy drinks almost never come up. Although the data presented at this workshop suggest that energy drinks have been replacing other sources of caffeine over the past few years, he has not been observing that trend. Most of his patients drink sweet tea, Mountain Dew, and occasionally Pepsi. Saul generally recommends moderation, which he considers 3–5 mg per kg per day, so 2 to 3 servings of 1 to 1.5 mg per kg.

With respect to the sudden deaths, Saul opined that almost all adolescents who die suddenly have an underlying cardiac condition. Not all conditions can be identified, but they include long QT syndrome, hypertrophic cardiomyopathy, arrhythmogenic right ventricular dysplasia, and catecholaminergic polymorphic ventricular tachycardia. Although one might expect individuals with any of these underlying conditions to be sensitive to caffeine, the evidence does not indicate such.

JOHN R. WHITE, JR., Pharm.D., WASHINGTON STATE UNIVERSITY, SPOKANE

John White commented on a suggestion made earlier during the workshop that the rapid intake of caffeine associated with energy drink consumption is problematic. In his opinion, however, based on the kinetics of caffeine, that is, time of absorption and half-life, intake time is of only nominal consequence with respect to peak concentrations. On the basis of some models that he has run, White observed that peak concentrations are the same whether the input is immediate (intravenous), fast (5 minutes), or slow (45 minutes). White also commented on the association between caffeine and risky behavior and cautioned that there are not enough data to suggest a causal relationship between the consumption of caffeinated energy drinks and progression to the use of more-addictive drugs.

REFERENCES

Bronstein, A. C., D. A. Spyker, L. R. Cantilena, B. H. Rumack, and R. C. Dart. 2011. 2011 annual report of the American Association of Poison Control Centers' National Poison Data Systems (NPDS): 29th annual report. *Clinical Toxicology* 50:911–1164.

Frassica, J. J., E. J. Orav, E. P. Walsh, and S. E. Lipshultz. 1994. Arrhythmias in children prenatally exposed to cocaine. *Archives of Pediatric and Adolescent Medicine* 148(11):1163–1169.

Lipshultz, S. E. 2000. Ventricular dysfunction clinical research in infants, children and adolescents. *Progress in Pediatric Cardiology* 12(1):1–28.

Seifert, S. M., J. L. Schaechter, E. R. Hershorin, and S. E. Lipshultz. 2011. Health effects of energy drinks on children, adolescents, and youth. *Pediatrics* 127(3):511–528.

9

Moving Forward: Filling the Data Gaps

Other than certain nutrients, probably no other food ingredient has been more heavily studied than caffeine. Yet, as illustrated throughout this report, a wealth of unanswered questions remains about exposure to caffeine in food and dietary supplements and the health consequences of that exposure, especially in certain potentially vulnerable populations (e.g., children, adolescents, individuals with underlying genetic susceptibilities, pregnant women). Indeed, this workshop was convened in part to identify major data gaps.

Throughout the workshop, individual speakers mentioned relevant data gaps. Jennifer Temple, in Chapter 6, thought the current data on energy drink usage among children and adolescents was out of date. Furthermore, she identified a need for prospective research relating the early use of caffeine to subsequent substance abuse. She also asked for research on the long-term effects of caffeine use, particularly among vulnerable groups. Also in Chapter 6, Amelia Arria noted a lack of valid assessment methods for energy drink consumption as a data gap, and she reinforced her comments in the final workshop session.

In the final session of the workshop, panelists identified what they each considered the most important data gaps and considered ways to fill those gaps. This chapter summarizes the panelists' presentations and the discussion that followed. Note that here, as throughout this report, the observations and opinions expressed are those of individual workshop participants.

Before the panelists spoke, moderator Joseph V. Rodricks, Ph.D., Environ, categorized potential data gaps into five major categories: (1) acute and chronic adverse health effects of caffeine; (2) dose–response issues requiring further study; (3) population variability and how dose–response relationships vary among populations; (4) interactions among ingredients in products that contain caffeine; and (5) intake and exposure issues requiring further study. Box 9-1 describes key points made by the speakers.

BOX 9-1
Key Points Made by Individual Speakers

- Amelia Arria suggested that more systematic data collection is needed to better understand patterns of caffeine use over time. Arria suggested that the variable methods used to assess caffeine exposure may partially explain some surveys' disparate findings (e.g., different findings regarding substitution versus addition of different sources of caffeine). She also suggested developing a more proactive approach to evaluating the magnitude of health consequences associated with caffeine use and developing screening tools that busy physicians can use to estimate the proportion of cardiovascular cases potentially attributable to caffeinated energy drink use.
- According to Alvin Bronstein, the national poison call center database lends itself to more systematic data collection and analysis. Acknowledging the nuanced nature of the data, Bronstein encouraged workshop participants to consider the many untapped ways that the data could be used. He also suggested that educating the public about the existence of poison call centers and that changing the name of the centers by replacing the word "poison" with a less alarming word might help to alleviate underreporting.
- Regan Bailey raised another semantics issue, that is, the use of the term "energy drink." She noted that many energy products in the dietary supplement label database do not contain caffeine. She urged that the words "caffeine" and "energy" not be used synonymously when discussing energy drinks or other energy products.
- Bailey identified the lack of data on the amount of caffeine in caffeine-containing foods and dietary supplements as the most critical data gap. Not having those data make it difficult to assess exposure.
- Christina Chambers added that among pregnant women, a critical data gap is exposure levels in the period of time prior to pregnancy recognition. Chambers advocated for cohort studies to help fill that and other data gaps.
- Steven Lipshultz said that when safety signals emerge, it is difficult to know who is at risk, the percentage of individuals at risk, or the severity of the risk. Lipshultz explained how this is true of any safety signal and emphasized the importance of the well-designed clinical study as a means to addressing these questions.
- On the basis of what has been reported thus far in the scientific literature, Stephen Schaffer called for more data on both the acute and chronic effects of combinations of ingredients in caffeinated energy drinks.

PANELIST REMARKS

Amelia M. Arria, Ph.D.
University of Maryland, College Park

Although caffeine has been widely studied and is well understood, Amelia Arria emphasized the need for more data on new ways that new caffeine-containing products are being consumed. Specifically, she called for estimates of the prevalence of use and possible health hazards associated with that use.

Arria suggested that the varying methods used to assess caffeine exposure may partially explain some surveys' disparate findings. She observed that data presented during the workshop from the International Life Sciences Institute (ILSI) and National Health and Nutrition Examination Survey (NHANES) analyses did not inform about the proportion of the population who used caffeine in the past month or past year, which are standard items that would be captured in other federally sponsored surveillance systems (see Chapter 2 for a summary of the ILSI and NHANES analyses presented at this workshop). She urged leveraging opportunities from what she identified as the most widely used survey of American school children, the National Institutes of Health (NIH)-sponsored "Monitoring the Future" survey, which began asking about energy drinks in 2010. As far as she was aware, the only publicly reported results from that survey were in a 2011 press release stating that the results indicated recent use among 35 percent of 8th graders and 29 percent of 10th and 12th graders.

In addition, Arria called for a better understanding of the proportion of children with underlying cardiovascular medical conditions who are being exposed to high levels of caffeine. Such an understanding will help to gauge the public health response. In response to physicians in the workshop audience who had indicated at various times during the discussion that none of their patients were attributing their medical complaints to energy drinks, Arria asked in return, "How systematically are you asking about recent consumption of energy drinks when a patient, especially an adolescent patient, presents with cardiovascular symptoms?" Better assessment and screening tools for busy physicians are needed to estimate the true proportion of cases that can be attributable to energy drink use. For Arria, the "bottom line" with respect to data methods is the need to start asking and reporting more systematically by putting forms into the hands of physicians who see patients with cardiovascular complications. It is a classic problem in epidemiologic surveillance, one analogous to parents' reports of children's alcohol consumption. Arria said, "They don't ask. Children don't tell."

Regarding the substitution of different sources of caffeine, Arria mentioned data suggesting that, contrary to what was suggested earlier in the workshop, energy drinks in young adults are being consumed in addition to, rather than instead of, traditional caffeinated beverages. Specifically, her own data from approximately one thousand young adults in their fourth year of college showed that 3.4 percent did not use any form of caffeine; 2.6 percent used energy drinks but no coffee, tea, or soda; 31 percent used coffee, soda, or tea but no energy drinks; and 63 percent used both energy drinks and another type of caffeinated beverage (Arria, 2013).

Arria commented on evaluations of the magnitude of health consequences associated with caffeine use. Many evaluations rely on what she described as "tip of the iceberg" datasets that measure only the most severe consequences. Federally sponsored surveillance of emergency department admissions, poison control, and the U.S. Food and Drug Administration's (FDA's) Adverse Event Reporting System are some examples, although many people are not even aware that they can call poison control centers or that the FDA has this reporting system. Although these datasets are useful for providing safety signals of what might be below the surface, they hugely underestimate the true proportion of medical complications that might be associated with the consumption of any one substance. A preferable approach to estimating the proportion of individuals experiencing health problems would be to ask consumers proactively about their experiences, an approach akin to the required and rigorous methods for adverse event reporting for pharmaceuticals in clinical trials.

Finally, said Arria, other data gaps include the safety among adolescents of current product formulations involving higher doses; interactions between caffeine and other ingredients, including medications; the use of highly caffeinated beverages before and during exercise, especially with young people; and basic data on the pharmacokinetics of caffeine under different circumstances of consumption, such as hot versus cold, and among individuals with varying sensitivities or genetic differences.

Alvin C. Bronstein, M.D., FACEP

Rocky Mountain Poison Center, Denver, Colorado

Alvin Bronstein discussed how poison centers can help to address some of the many unanswered questions about how these caffeine-containing products are used, whether any health issues are associated with their use, and which populations are most at risk. He proposed that researchers look more closely at poison center data. He and his colleagues have focused on single exposures, but the poison center database lends itself to mixed exposures as well—for example, when people use a product in combination with ethanol or another drug. Bronstein recognized the nuances of poison center data and the need to interpret them carefully, but he emphasized the systematized way that those data can be gathered.

With respect to underreporting and ways to encourage more people to call poison centers to report issues with products, Bronstein suggested that perhaps the word "poison" needs to be replaced. The public also needs to be educated that such centers are places where one can call to talk to a health care professional.

In addition to a data resource, poison centers also function as a surveillance system for identifying index cases and cases that meet certain syndromic surveillance criteria.

Regan L. Bailey, Ph.D., R.D.
Office of Dietary Supplements, National Institutes of Health, Bethesda, Maryland

The first gap that needs to be filled, in Regan Bailey's opinion, is to define "energy product." She observed that "caffeine" and "energy" seem to be used synonymously, but they are not the same. Many energy products in the dietary supplement label database contain no caffeine at all and are simply high-dose B vitamins. Approximately 1,500 products in the dietary supplement label database have energy listed somewhere on the label, and 157 products have "energy" in the product name. Some of those products have caffeine, and others do not.

Another important need pointed out by Bailey is a database on the amount of caffeine in caffeine-containing foods and dietary supplements. Although caffeine must be listed on a label if a product contains caffeine, the amount of caffeine present is not required. Not having that information makes it difficult to assess usual intakes of caffeine and to assess usage patterns.

It is not even clear at this point how best to assess usage, Bailey said. Social desirability issues may impact reporting, for example, with children not telling their parents that they are using caffeinated products or with people feeling embarrassed that they are using them. Also, beverages are often forgotten foods in reporting on 24-hour recalls or other types of dietary assessment methods. Although NHANES serves as a good tool for monitoring, it might not be the best method for answering some questions. That said, Bailey has used NHANES data to examine energy drink use from two 24-hour recalls. People who had used a product on either of those two occasions were considered "users." Given that definition, from 2007 to 2010, 2 percent of the U.S. population were users. Energy drink use was most common in males from 19 to 30 years of age, with 5 percent of that population defined as users. The most common product used was Red Bull, providing an average of 154 mg caffeine per day.

Christina Chambers, Ph.D., M.D.
University of California, San Diego

Christina Chambers reiterated that although there is quite a bit of data on low to moderate caffeine consumption in pregnant women, there are less data on high-dose exposure to traditional caffeine-containing products (i.e., coffee, tea, and cola) and no data on newer caffeine-containing products. An important period of time to consider measuring or better measuring the effects of these exposure levels is prior to pregnancy recognition.

Chambers called for improved methods to estimate both acute and chronic exposure. She agreed with Bailey that dietary recalls may not capture everything and wondered about the potential to develop a technology that might be more continuous or at least repeated through the course of pregnancy, or any period of time, to capture other than a snapshot of information.

Another knowledge gap is in the area of health behaviors surrounding caffeine consumption, particularly high levels of consumption, and whether those behaviors are associated with any other risky behaviors. Chambers opined that a cohort approach would be the optimal way to collect that type of information. One of the major benefits of the survey design of the National Children's Study, as it was originally proposed, is its ability to collect this kind of information on a very large sample of women and their children over the course of a pregnancy.

Steven E. Lipshultz, M.D.
University of Miami, Florida

After spending 35 years looking at first-generation survivors of many formerly fatal illnesses of early childhood and seeing late effects after transient early exposures to chemotherapy, Steven Lipshultz has learned that he and his colleagues do not really know when safety signals come up, who is at risk, what percentage of their patients are at risk, or the degree of severity. For example, about 1 percent of childhood cancer survivors experience acute heart failure, which is the leading late effect for early exposure, especially for those who were exposed early in life. Physicians are seeing the same effect with early-in-life exposure to antiretroviral therapy to block transmission. Radiation exposure is another type of exposure with long-term consequences. Lipshultz and colleagues recently published a paper on the follow-up of 18 million patients who had received radiation and found a strong signal for heart disease.

It is a recurring theme, Lipshultz observed, that exposures have long-term consequences. Still, even when a safety signal, or something that might be a safety signal, is detected in a vulnerable population, such as in children, it may be only the tip of the iceberg. Lipshultz said, "It might be true. It might not. It might be important. It might not."

An appropriate study design is essential for this type of long-term study, given that one cannot think a priori of all the questions that might come up. His approach is to let the patients direct what is necessary. He usually approaches the design in three ways. First, he gains an understanding of the clinical course. In order to gain continuous funding for a lifetime-exposure-effects study, one needs unambiguous quantitative subclinical data. Second, he identifies risk factors, whether those are whole exosome sequences, biomarkers, or something else. Third, as part of the longitudinal study, he evaluates whether any of what he had initially identified as theoretically vulnerable populations are truly of concern.

Lipshultz observed that many of his colleagues make recommendations on the basis of clinical impression. For him, the question is, "How do we go from clinical impression to understanding where the truth is?" The answer: only by conducting a longitudinal study and determining whether any of the risk biomarkers are truly predictive of outcome based on a higher incidence of subclinical or, later, clinical issues.

Stephen Schaffer, Ph.D.
University of South Alabama, Mobile

When looking through the scientific literature on ingredients in caffeinated energy drinks, Stephen Schaffer was struck by how little literature there was. When attempting to define the interactions of the various ingredients in such drinks, he found basically no information at either the animal or human level about the effects of such interactions on either cardiovascular or central nervous system physiology. The clinical studies that have been reported were not conducted properly, in his opinion, with very few randomized, double-blind, well-controlled studies.

In addition, he emphasized the need to study both acute and chronic exposure, given that chronic exposure can alter gene regulation and that responses to chronic exposure can be very different from responses to acute exposure. He also urged consideration of how energy drinks affect energy metabolism, blood glucose levels, and insulin secretion. Finally, many energy drink ingredients are antioxidants. Although antioxidants are generally perceived as good, some scientists now argue that too many antioxidants can be problematic. In sum, Schaffer said, "There's a lot of work to be done."

In addition to better defining the science, Schaffer called for defining what a vulnerable population is. What is the evidence that a vulnerable group is vulnerable? "If you can't provide the scientific evidence [that] they are vulnerable groups," he said, "you don't have vulnerable groups."

PANELIST DISCUSSION WITH THE AUDIENCE

In the final panelist discussion with the audience, most questions asked of the panelists revolved around the differences between a longitudinal follow-up study and a registry, both of which were suggested at various times over the course of the workshop; the pros and cons of taking the sort of approach that Health Canada has taken with respect to setting safety standards for potentially vulnerable populations; other types of potential safety signals worth evaluating (i.e., besides sudden cardiac death); the potential value of data from military studies on caffeine exposure; and the potential value of industry data and the availability of such data. This section summarizes the discussion that took place.

What Next?: Longitudinal Follow-Up Study, Registry, or Something Else?

Lipshultz and Bronstein were asked to clarify the different roles that a longitudinal study and registry would serve with respect to tracking and analyzing potential safety signals associated with caffeine-containing foods and dietary supplements. Lipshultz replied that the two types of research are very different.

Generally, registries provide a means to understand the course of exposure and characterize the exposed population. That information can then be used to formulate any of a number of hypotheses about that exposure. Lipshultz noted that, in addition to designing and conducting longitudinal studies, he has been the principal investigator of the National Heart, Lung, and Blood Institute (NHLBI) Pediatric Cardiomyopathy Registry for more than three decades. The registry, which was set up as a way to collect more consistent outcomes for children with cardiomyopathies, helped researchers better understand the course of outcomes and identify potential risk factors. Lipshultz described it as "a very useful platform." Later, NHLBI decided to also fund a biological specimen laboratory, which the researchers have been using to see whether some patients are more genetically susceptibility to poor outcomes. He and his colleagues recently published a paper demonstrating a ninefold increased rate of dead heart muscle with certain exposures. Lynn Goldman noted that an additional value of registries is that their large size allows for rare effects to be studied.

Lipshultz explained that longitudinal cohort studies, on the other hand, are more hypothesis-driven. They are more limited in scope, with very select inclusion and exclusion criteria based on what is known about likely risk. They are the type of study conducted when a safety signal exists and needs to be tested.

Either way, according to Lipshultz, whether one embarks with a registry or longitudinal study, 5 years from now the field is going to be in a much better position to answer many of the questions being put forth at this workshop. With a cohort study, some questions will be answered. With a registry, exposed patients will be better characterized.

He emphasized the lack of consensus around safety concerns associated with caffeine-containing products. He said, "Your degree of concern varies based on who you are in this room." Nonetheless, there are concerns. Given those concerns, in his opinion the next step is to evaluate those concerns, whether through a registry or a longitudinal cohort study. They are both potentially valuable designs.

Bronstein clarified that he had not recommended a registry per se. Rather, he was recommending that poison center data be used to answer many of the questions being put forth at this workshop—for example, questions about caffeine consumption in combination with other ingredients or caffeinated product consumption in combination with other products. In addition to reporting exposures, the poison center's current surveillance system could be expanded from tracking exposures in real time to evaluating exposures on a weekly or even daily basis. Trends could be identified, and cases that meet certain public health criteria could be investigated. As an example of how poison center data have been used in the past, he mentioned a product called Total Body Formula, a dietary supplement product that contained excess selenium, which caused, among other effects, nail changes and hair loss. The FDA removed the product from the market. Poison centers worked with the FDA and the CDC to locate the approximately 160 cases called to poison centers so that public health departments could investigate the cases. He reiterated that the public needs to be better educated about poison centers.

Goldman noted that many people for many years have believed that the poison center reporting/surveillance system could be improved with more complete case follow-up, not just for caffeine- and energy drink–related calls but for many other types of calls as well. Goldman noted the difficulty in interpreting a lot of poison center data because of the lack of data on outcomes.

Health Canada's Approach to Setting Safety Standards for Caffeine Exposure

Given so many uncertainties in the science of the safety of caffeine-containing foods and beverages, Health Canada, in Goldman's opinion, seems to have taken what she described as "kind of a simple approach" by advising healthy people to consume no more than 400 mg per day, pregnant women to consume no more than 300 mg per day, and children to consume no more than 2.5 mg per kg per day. Although this advice is pragmatic in terms of what is known and what is not known about safe levels of caffeine exposure, is it an appropriate approach?

Steven Lipshultz replied that the levels are based on the best available population data. In his opinion, although population data and population-based recommendations are important, this approach may not be an appropriate one for specific vulnerable groups, whether those groups are defined as such on the basis of research or clinician concern. When potentially vulnerable populations are identified, the typical pediatric approach is to determine safe levels in those populations and, at the same time, avoid exposure if there is no real therapeutic efficacy associated with such exposure. Rodricks clarified that the Health Canada recommendation is not a single standard and that it includes two recognized vulnerable populations, women of childbearing age and children. Even so, Lipshultz said, among children there are potentially vulnerable subpopulations—for example, children with cardiomyopathies and arrhythmias. For those children, is the standard for all children appropriate? He said, "I bet you would find almost no pediatric cardiologist that would buy into that concept. If you think there are vulnerable populations, it behooves you to either protect them, test it, or do both."

While agreeing with Lipshultz, Arria opined that recommendations are among the weakest public health responses and that more effective risk management will require a stronger response. People do things other than what is recommended. Chambers agreed, noting that most women interpret "reproductive age" as "when I am pregnant." Not only does the evidence need to support that all women of reproductive age, pregnant or not, are at increased risk for adverse outcomes; another issue to consider is whether the adverse outcome(s) of concern even matters to individual patients. For example, some women and health care providers may not consider the risk of delivering a baby 50 grams lighter than the infant would be otherwise to be an important risk.

For Schaffer, the problem (with making recommendations for vulnerable populations) is that "the science isn't there." When someone dies a sudden death or develops an arrhythmia, one can look back in history and determine that the patient consumed some energy drinks. But there are no double-blind, randomized studies where different groups of individuals consume different combinations of energy drinks or other products and an end point is examined. "That's the problem," he said. "Until you define clearly what the vulnerable groups are and under what conditions, then I think it's very difficult to make recommendations." Rodricks replied that the Health Canada recommendations are in fact based on a large number of studies. Schaffer opined that more studies need to be done. He said, "Carefully controlled studies need to be done to define what a vulnerable group is—if there is in fact a vulnerable group and under what conditions."

Arria agreed that if the ability existed to do those randomized controlled trials, questions would be answered. But conducting such trials would be difficult given ethical concerns about administering doses similar to what are being consumed in the natural population, particularly doses being consumed by adolescents and young adults. She said, "I don't think you could get it through an investigative review board (IRB) to randomly assign children and adolescents and even young adults to high doses of caffeine." The type of naturalistic cohort study described by Lipshultz, on the other hand, where high doses are not administered but rather natural levels of consumption are measured, would be advantageous in that regard.

Other Potential Safety Signals

In Roland Griffiths's opinion, one of the safety signals for which the most data have been produced is physical dependence. While many other adverse effect signals are difficult to study, with ethical constraints limiting prospective research, physical dependence has not been similarly constrained. Researchers have learned quite a bit about physical dependence from prospective studies. Although it is not as serious as sudden death, neither is it a trivial issue. An exposure level as low as 100 mg per day is enough to produce headache. As a parent, Griffiths said that he would not want his children to be erratically going in and out of caffeine withdrawal while attending school and trying to learn. It is known that a withdrawal signal exists in doses that are relatively low, low enough to be detectable in a single can of many energy drinks. He suggested that further consideration be given to restraining the promotion of those products to school-age children.

The Value and Availability of Military Data

A member of the audience asked whether any data being collected by the military might be helpful, given that both energy drink and caffeine consumption in the military are quite high and that an Institute of Medicine Committee on Military Nutrition Research has issued a few reports on caffeine consumption over the years. There was some agreement among the panelists that this was a good suggestion. Chambers noted that the U.S. Millennium Cohort Study is following families with active-duty military family members and that it would be a good way to study exposure to caffeine-containing products.

The Value and Availability of Industry Data

Although some physicians have not seen the signals that others are seeing, John Higgins observed that, nonetheless, signals are being seen and should not be ignored. At the very least, more information should be gathered. Are the signals real, or are they an artifact? He called for more research, specifically research on caffeine-containing energy drinks. He said, "The signals we are hearing are from these beverages, not from caffeine, not from coffee." He recognized the challenge and questioned whether any of the manufacturers might be able to help by providing marketing and testing data. Marketing data could help researchers to understand exposure (who is being exposed), and testing data could help them to understand the effects of consumption.

Bob Arnot, representing Monster Energy, responded by clarifying that the company decided not to market their product to children because of a lack of safety data. He observed that the label on the can states the product is not recommended for children, pregnant women, or sensitive populations. In addition, all cans are labeled with the amount of caffeine. He acknowledged the contentiousness of the issue with regard to adolescents and observed that the company does not market to adolescents. For example, they do not advertise on top-40 radio or through television. Arnot observed that company leadership is as concerned about the issue as the scientific community is and is looking as actively. "They haven't seen anything," he said. He remarked that when the American Medical Association issued its warning about energy drinks, they did so under the assumption that energy drinks have 50 times as much caffeine as coffee. One of the surprises about mainstream energy drinks is how little caffeine they contain. An 8-ounce serving contains roughly 80 mg of caffeine, whereas a commercial coffee product has 320 mg of caffeine. On a milligram-per-ounce basis, energy drinks have half the caffeine of coffee.

Later during the discussion, Arnot communicated that he had been in touch with company leadership and that they were happy to enter a dialogue.

Lipshultz applauded the idea of partnering among industry, the FDA, and others. He observed that about 17 years ago, when he was a voting member on the FDA Oncologic Drugs Advisory Committee, some terrible cardiac signals associated with a prescription product emerged but that there was inadequate data to study those signals. The company involved agreed to participate with the FDA and to conduct studies to gather the necessary data, so a black box warning label was issued. Several years later, postmarket surveillance indicated that the signals were still present, but the promised research was never delivered. Over the past several years, similar issues have come up with over-the-counter products for children. Although he applauded industry's willingness to at least consider providing data, he questioned what to do in the meantime given that there is no life-saving therapeutic reason to consume these products and that multiple independent databases have yielded safety signals. In his opinion, until safety is established, it is important to consider how to move forward in the meantime.

REFERENCE

Arria, A. M. 2013 (unpublished). *The college life study*. http://www.cls.umd.edu (accessed December 5, 2013).

A

Workshop Agenda

Caffeine in Food and Dietary Supplements: Examining Safety

Planning Committee on Potential Health Hazards Associated with Consumption of Caffeine in Food and Dietary Supplements

The National Academies Lecture Room
2101 Constitution Avenue NW
Washington, DC 20418

August 5–6, 2013

WORKSHOP OBJECTIVES

- Evaluate the epidemiological, toxicological, clinical, and other relevant literature to describe important health hazards associated with caffeine consumption
- Delineate vulnerable populations who may be at risk from caffeine exposure
- Describe caffeine exposure and risk of cardiovascular and other health effects on vulnerable populations, including additive effects with other ingredients and effects related to preexisting conditions
- Explore safe caffeine exposure levels for general and vulnerable populations
- Identify data gaps on caffeine stimulant effects including but not limited to cardiovascular, central nervous system, or other health outcomes

August 5, 2013

8:00–8:45 a.m. **Registration**

INTRODUCTION AND OPENING REMARKS

8:50 a.m. **Welcome**
Lynn Goldman, George Washington University, Chair, Planning Committee on Potential Health Hazards Associated with Consumption of Caffeine in Food and Dietary Supplements

9:00 a.m. **Opening Remarks**
Margaret Hamburg, Commissioner of Food and Drugs, Food and Drug Administration

SESSION 1: INTAKE AND EXPOSURE TO CAFFEINE

Moderated by Barbara Petersen, Exponent

9:15 a.m. **Examining Exposure to Caffeine in Foods, Beverage, and Supplements**

Caffeine Intakes from Beverages in the United States
Diane Mitchell, Penn State University

Trends in Caffeine Consumption
Victor Fulgoni III, Nutrition Impact, LLC

10:00 a.m. **Panel Discussion with Speakers**

10:30 a.m. **Break**

SESSION 2: SAFETY SIGNALS AND SURVEILLANCE OF POPULATIONS

Moderated by Steve Lipshultz, University of Miami

10:50 a.m. **Type and Frequency of Caffeine Toxicity: U.S. and International Surveillance**
Alvin Bronstein, Rocky Mountain Poison Center

11:10 a.m. **Safety Assessment of Caffeine in Foods and Beverages**
Ashley Roberts, Intertek Cantox Consulting (by WebEx)

11:30 a.m. **Panel Discussion with Speakers**

12:00 p.m. **Break for Lunch**

SESSION 3: CAFFEINE EFFECTS ON THE CARDIOVASCULAR SYSTEM

Moderated by Stephen Daniels, Children's Hospital, University of Colorado, Denver

1:00 p.m. **Vascular Effects of Caffeine**
John Higgins, University of Texas Medical School

1:20 p.m. **Caffeine and Risk of Arrhythmia**
Jeffrey Goldberger, Northwestern University

1:40 p.m. **Caffeine and Risk of Hypertension**
Ahmed El-Sohemy, University of Toronto (by WebEx)

2:00 p.m. **Panel Discussion with Speakers**

SESSION 4: CAFFEINE EFFECTS ON THE CENTRAL NERVOUS SYSTEM

Moderated by Thomas Gould, Temple University

2:20 p.m.	**Neuropharmacologic Effects of Caffeine Exposure** *Sergi Ferré, National Institutes of Health, National Institute on Drug Abuse*
2:40 p.m.	**Developmental Neurological Effects of Caffeine Exposure** *Jennifer Temple, University of Buffalo (by WebEx)*
3:00 p.m.	**Panel Discussion with Speakers**
3:20 p.m.	**Break**

SESSION 5: PANEL DISCUSSION: BEHAVIORAL EFFECTS ASSOCIATED WITH CAFFEINE CONSUMPTION

Moderated by Richard Adamson, TPN Associates

3:30 p.m.	**Dependence/Tolerance** *Roland Griffiths, Johns Hopkins University*
	Addiction *Charles O'Brien, University of Pennsylvania*
	Risk Taking *Amelia Arria, University of Maryland, College Park*
4:30 p.m.	**Public Comments**

PUBLIC COMMENTS AND CONCLUDING REMARKS

5:00 p.m. **Concluding Remarks for Day 1**
Lynn Goldman, George Washington University, Chair, Planning Committee on Potential Health Hazards Associated with Consumption of Caffeine in Food and Dietary Supplements

5:10 p.m. **Adjourn Meeting**

August 6, 2013

8:50 a.m. **Welcome and Summary from Day 1**
Lynn Goldman, George Washington University, Chair, Planning Committee on Potential Health Hazards Associated with Consumption of Caffeine in Food and Dietary Supplements

9:00 a.m. **Opening Remarks**
Michael Taylor, Deputy Commissioner for Foods and Veterinary Medicine, Food and Drug Administration

SESSION 1: OTHER COMPOUNDS IMPACTING CAFFEINE EFFECTS

Moderated by James Coughlin, Coughlin & Associates

9:15 a.m. **Facilitated Discussion: Other Components Impacting Caffeine Effects**
Led by Stephen Schaffer, University of South Alabama

Summary of the Issues
Stephen Schaffer

Panel Discussion
Speakers from Day 1

SESSION 2: USE OF CAFFEINATED PRODUCTS

Moderated by: James Coughlin, Coughlin & Associates

10:15 a.m. **Trends in Usage and Potential Benefits from Caffeine**
Andrew Smith, Cardiff University, UK (by WebEx)

10:35 a.m. **Q&A**

SESSION 3: EXPLORING SAFE CAFFEINE EXPOSURE LEVELS

10:45 a.m. **Panel Discussion: Exploring Safe Caffeine Exposure Levels for Vulnerable Populations**

Panel Moderator
Mark Feeley, Health Canada

Pregnancy/Infants
Christina Chambers, University of California, San Diego

Children/ Young Adults
Steve Lipshultz, University of Miami

11:30 a.m. **Break for Lunch**

SESSION 4: DATA GAPS

Moderated by Joe Rodricks, Environ International

12:30 p.m. **Panel Discussion on Data Gaps and Future Research**
Stephen Schaffer, University of South Alabama
Christina Chambers, University of California, San Diego

Steve Lipshultz, University of Miami
Regan Bailey, National Institutes of Health, Office of Dietary Supplements
Amelia Arria, University of Maryland, College Park
Alvin Bronstein, Rocky Mountain Poison Center

1:45 p.m. **Chair's Summary and Final Thoughts**

Lynn Goldman, George Washington University, Chair, Planning Committee on Potential Health Hazards Associated with Consumption of Caffeine in Food and Dietary Supplements

2:00 p.m. **Adjourn Meeting**

B

Workshop Attendees

Naman Ahluwalia
Centers for Disease Control and Prevention

Rend Al-Mondhiry
Council for Responsible Nutrition

Joan Apgar
The Hershey Co.

Steven Armstrong
Campbell Soup Co.

Bob Arnot
Monster Energy Co.

Arti Arora
The Coca-Cola Co.

MaryJoy Ballantyne
Covington & Burling

James Bangasser
American Beverage Association (ABA)

Patrizia Barone
Unilever

Maureen Beach
ABA

Stephanie Beasley
Inside Health Policy

Michael Beckelic
Meda Consumer Healthcare Inc.

Nadine Bewry
U.S. Department of Food and Drug Administration (FDA)

Heidi Bialk
PepsiCo, Inc.

Sonya Billiard
Health Canada

Hope Bilyk
Rosalind Franklin University of Medicine and Science

Adrienne Black
Grocery Manufacturers Association (GMA)

Stephen Boehm
Purdue University

Michael Bolger
Exponent

Sarah Botha
Federal Trade Commission

Trudi Boyd
Story Partners

Rosalind Breslow
National Institutes of Health (NIH)

Lauren Brookmire
FDA

Whitney Brown
Academy of Nutrition and Dietetics (AND)

Jen Brulc
General Mills, Inc.

Leon Bruner
GMA

Brittany Bugbee
University of Maryland

Shelly Burgess
FDA

Robert Burns
GMA

Kaitlyn Buss
Story Partners

Kathryn Camp
NIH

Jessica Campbell
General Mills, Inc.

Susan Carlson
FDA

Murray Carpenter
Freelance

Kellie Casavale
U.S. Department of Health and Human Services (HHS)

Bruce Charash

Sonya Clay
American Academy of Pediatrics

Amy Clewell
AIBMR Life Sciences, Inc.

Ashley Cook
Health Canada

Michele Corash
Morrison & Foerster LLP

Mark Corey
Green Mountain Coffee Roasters, Inc.

Heather Nelson Cortes
Optimum Nutrition

Jaclyn Crouch
NIH

Cindy Davis
NIH

Tom Davis
Monster Energy Co.

Paul Dechary
Monster Energy Co.

Brady Dennis
Washington Post

Joseph DeRupo
National Coffee Association

Patricia Deuster
Uniformed Services University of the Health Sciences (USUHS)

Candace Doepker
ToxStrategies, Inc.

George Dunaif
GMA

Johanna Dwyer
NIH

Robert Earl
The Coca-Cola Co.

Marianne Smith Edge
IFIC

Anna Edney
Bloomberg

Theresa Eisenman
FDA

Dave Ellis
SportsRD

John Endres
AIBMR Life Sciences, Inc.

Cecilia Wilkinson Enns
U.S. Department of Agriculture (USDA)

Ilene Eskenazi

Daniel Fabricant
FDA

Suzanne Fitzpatrick
FDA

Jennifer Folliard
Academy of Nutrition and Dietetics

Michael Forman
MHFEDMD, Inc.

Ellen Fried
New York State Attorney General's Office

Joel Geerling
Harvard Medical School

Francesca Gessber
San Francisco City Attorney

Kevin Goldberg

Mark Gottlieb
Northeastern University

Amanda Grady
FDA

James Griffiths
CRN-International

Michael Gruber
GMA

Miriam Guggenheim
Covington & Burling LLP

Tracey Halliday
ABA

Amy Hancock
ABA

Eileen Harley
The Hershey Co.

Molly Harry
FDA

Aubri Hazlett
J.M. Smucker Co.

Alix Heard
Office of Rep. Frank Pallone

Kasey Heintz
FDA

Eric Hentges
International Life Sciences Institute (ILSI)

Steve Hertzler
Abbott Nutrition

Regina Hildwine
GMA

Nicole Hines
International Food Information Council (IFIC)

Elinor Hitchner
Bayer HealthCare

Sue Hite
Military Contractor

Jason Hlywka
Kraft Foods, Inc.

Rebecca Holmes
Red Bull North America

Judy Hong
Goldman Sachs

Joe Hovermill
Miles & Stockbridge

Terry Hughes
Monster Energy Co.

Brokini Ibukunola
Super Expedite Contractors Ltd.

Mark Itzkoff
Olsson Frank Weeda Terman Matz PC

Michael Jacobson
Center for Science in the Public Interest (CSPI)

David Jaffe
APCO Worldwide

Sumitha Jagadibabu
SIET College for Women

Diana Jeffery
Daniel Johnston

Donnamaria Jones
USUHS

Nicholas Kadysh

Saad Kamal
Washington Analysis

Mark Kantor
FDA

Subhashini Katumuluwa
NIH

Wanda Kelker
The Coca-Cola Co.

Brian Kennedy
GMA

Gerry Khermouch
Beverage Business Insights

Chor San Khoo
IFIC

Rick Kingston
University of Minnesota

Barbara Kochanowski
Consumer Healthcare Products Association

Nicole Kostelnick
Campbell Soup Co.

Alison Kretser
ILSI

Steve Kuo
Taipei Economic and Cultural Representative Office

Dorothy Lagg
Mars, Inc.

Barbara Larkin
Kellogg's

Jae Lee
Morrison & Foerster LLP

Ji-Eun Lee
Kellogg's

Shannon Leeke
GMA

Lisa Lefferts
CSPI

DeAnn Liska
Kellogg's

Craig Llewellyn
The Coca-Cola Co.

Emilia Lonardo
GMA

Lindsey Loving
IFIC

Stefano Luccioli
FDA

Zhelin Luo
Washington University

Maricel Maffini
The Pew Charitable Trusts

James Mann
Newsmith

Padma Maruvada
NIH

Arlene Mathes-Scharf
Kashrut.com

Robert Mathews
Keller and Heckman

Antonia Mattia
FDA

Jason May
Rockstar, Inc.

Sharon Mayl
FDA

Aileen McGrath
San Francisco City Attorney's Office

Carolyn Meduski
Nestlé USA

Carla Mejia
U.S. Pharmacopeia (USP)

Jeremy Mihalov
FDA

Farida Mohamedshah
Institute of Food Technologists

Amber Mosher
HHS

Victoria Muldrow-Greene
Walgreens

Jeff Mundt
Hershey

Jay Murray
Murray & Associates

George Muscat
Campbell Soup Co.

John Mwangi
Starbucks Coffee Co.

Marianna Naum
FDA

Emily Newman
Sidley Austin LLP

Karlheinz Niederreiter
Red Bull GmbH

Inge Lise Nielsen
Bayer Consumer Care

Maria Fernanda Nunez
University of Toronto

Claudia Nunn
Burdock Group

Julie Obbagy
USDA

Hellen Oketch-Rabah
USP

Stephen Ostroff
FDA

Stuart Pape Patton
Boggs LLP

Jennifer Person-Whippo
Naval Supply Systems Command

Elyse Petroni
Story Partners

Laura Pillsbury
FDA

Rachel Poole
Temple University

Lauren Pratapas

Justin Prochnow
Greenberg Traurig

Lucy Reid
Coca-Cola North America

Amy Rinaldo
Oakland Law Group

Alberto Rivera-Rentas
NIH

Danielle Robertson
Beachbody

Bob Roehr
British Medical Journal

Sarah Romotsky
IFIC

Leah Rosenfeld
FDA

Lauren Rossen
Centers for Disease Control and Prevention (CDC)

Joel Rotstein
Health Canada

Sylvia Rowe
SR StrategyJaclyn Royer GMA

Marvin Rubin
Ohio Public Health Association

Allen Rudman
FDA

Helene Rutledge
AeroDesigns, Inc.

Kari Ryan
Kraft Foods

Rodney Sacks
Monster Beverage Corporation

Leila Saldanha
NIH

Kathleen Sanzo
Morgan Lewis & Bockius

Nandakumara Sarma
USP

Elyse Sartor
NIH

Phil Saul
University of South Carolina

Hilton Schlosberg
Monster Energy Co.

Marilyn Schorin
Schorin Strategics, LLC

Laura Shumow
National Confectioners Association

Jay Sirois
Certified Healthcare Protection Administrators

Kira Slagle
Optimum Health Solutions, Inc.

Rebecca Slater
Podesta Group

Kelly Smith
Dr Pepper Snapple Group

Rob Smith
Capital Alpha Partners

Meena Somanchi
USDA

Barbara Sorkin
NIH

Tara Steeley
Office of the City Attorney of San Francisco

Dan Steffen
A-D Policy Analysis

Mark Stephens
USUHS

Eve Essery Stoody
USDA

Melissa Stringfellow
FDA

Amy Sunderman
Reckitt Benckiser

Christine Swanson
NIH

Stanley Tarka
The Tarka Group, Inc.

Donna Thede
Kellogg's

Janet Thorlton
Purdue University

Lisa Thorsten
Campbell Soup Co.

Lorna Totman
Lorna Totman Consulting, LLC

Ken Trombetta
Hoplite Capital Management

Pepin Tuma
AND

Shashwat Udit
Broadwood Capital

Pat Vanderkooy
Dietitians of Canada

Patricia Vaughan
ABA

Laura Venker
Keller & Heckman, LLP

Marie Vicinanzo
Novartis Consumer Health

Tom Vollmuth
Wrigley, Inc.

Brian Waldman
Arent Fox LLP

Taylor Wallace
National Osteoporosis Foundation

Isabel Walls
USDA

Brenda Watson
Nestlé Nutrition Canada

Cara Welch
Natural Products Association

Ann Wennberg
Abbott Nutrition

Nancy Wesensten
Walter Reed Army Institute of Research

Alex Wohl
FDA

John White

Arthur Whitmore
FDA

Joe Wilson
UBS

Kimberly Wingfield
GMA

Nancy Yanish
FDA

Jeffrey Zhao
ILSI North America

Sam Zeller
Unilever

Gary Zizka
Olsson Frank Weeda Terman Matz PC

C

Biographical Sketches of Workshop Speakers and Moderators

SPEAKERS: OPENING REMARKS

Margaret A. Hamburg, M.D., is commissioner of the Food and Drug Administration (FDA), where she has served since May 2009. As FDA commissioner, she is advancing regulatory science, medical product innovation, and globalization of the agency while overseeing the implementation of groundbreaking laws to curb the use of tobacco and to enhance food safety. She has undertaken major efforts to streamline and modernize the FDA's regulatory pathways. Before joining the FDA, Dr. Hamburg was vice president and senior scientist at the Nuclear Threat Initiative. In the 1990s, as New York City's health commissioner, she launched several major initiatives, including the nation's first public health bioterrorism preparedness program and an internationally recognized program to curtail the resurgence and spread of tubercle bacillus. President Clinton later named her assistant secretary for planning and evaluation in the U.S. Department of Health and Human Services.

Michael R. Taylor, J.D., is deputy commissioner for foods and veterinary medicine at the FDA. In this position, he provides leadership and direction to the Center for Food Safety and Applied Nutrition and the Center for Veterinary Medicine. He also works closely with the foods-related programs of the FDA's inspection and compliance arm, the Office of Regulatory Affairs. Dr. Taylor is responsible for establishing a modern, science-based, and prevention-oriented food safety program for domestic and imported foods. He also leads such critical areas as food labeling, nutrition, animal drug safety and effectiveness, and scientific capacity. Dr. Taylor served previously in senior positions at the FDA and the U.S. Department of Agriculture, as a research professor in academia, and on several National Academy of Sciences (NAS) expert committees.

SPEAKERS

Amelia M. Arria, Ph.D., is associate professor of behavioral and community health and director of the Center on Young Adult Health and Development at the University of Maryland, College Park, School of Public Health. She is the principal investigator on the College Life Study, a 10-year longitudinal prospective study of college students. Dr. Arria has conducted research studies on adolescent and young adult health risk behaviors, including energy drink consumption patterns and the relationship between energy drink use and other forms of substance use. She is currently involved in several efforts to translate research findings for parents and policy makers.

Regan L. Bailey, Ph.D., R.D., is a nutritional epidemiologist in the Office of Dietary Supplements, Office of Disease Prevention, at the National Institutes of Health (NIH). Dr. Bailey is also the director of the annual Mary Frances Picciano Dietary Supplement Research Practicum and the director of career development and outreach. In addition, she is an adjunct professor in the Department of Foods and Nutrition at Purdue University. The overarching goal of her research program is to prevent or lessen the risk of chronic disease through nutrition. Dr. Bailey has considerable expertise working with the National Health and Nutrition Examination Survey. She is a member of the American Society for Nutrition and the Academy of Nutrition and Dietetics. She is also on the executive board of the Nutrition Epidemiology Research Interest Section of the American Society for Nutrition. She serves as an advisor to the International Life Sciences Institute–North America both on the Fortification Committee and in the Food, Nutrition and Safety Program. She is a registered dietitian.

Alvin C. Bronstein, M.D., is medical director of the Rocky Mountain Poison Center, the regional poison center for the states of Colorado, Hawaii, Montana, and Nevada. He is also associate professor in the Department of Emergency Medicine, University of Colorado School of Medicine. In addition to his responsibilities as medical director, Dr.

Bronstein actively participates in the poison center's medical toxicology training program, oversees toxicology training for the center's poison information specialists and providers, and directs the center's Continuous Quality Improvement program. His research interests include creating new methods to deliver poison information services using computer databases and poison center data surveillance and trend analysis.

Christina Chambers, Ph.D., M.P.H., is professor in the Department of Pediatrics, School of Medicine, and associate director of the Clinical and Translational Research Institute at the University of California, San Diego. She is a perinatal epidemiologist and teratologist who specializes in research related to the effects of prenatal and breastfeeding exposure to recreational substances, medications, vaccines, chemicals, and other environmental agents on the developing embryo, fetus, infant, or child.

Ahmed El-Sohemy, Ph.D., is associate professor in the Department of Nutritional Sciences and holds a Canada Research Chair in nutrigenomics. He is the founder of Nutrigenomix Inc. and serves as chief science officer. Dr. El-Sohemy joined the faculty at the University of Toronto in 2000 to establish a research program in nutrigenomics. The goal of his research is to identify biomarkers of dietary exposure and elucidate the genetic basis for variability in nutrient response and dietary preferences. He collaborates with researchers across Canada as well as the United States, Costa Rica, Denmark, Italy, Switzerland, South Korea, and Singapore. Dr. El-Sohemy has served on international expert advisory panels and scientific advisory boards of several organizations, and was appointed to Health Canada's Scientific Advisory Board.

Sergi Ferré, Ph.D., M.D., is senior investigator and chief of the Integrative Neurobiology Section at the National Institute on Drug Abuse Intramural Research Program. Dr. Ferré is interested in the role of receptor heteromers as targets for drug development in neuropsychiatric disorders and drug addiction. His research deals preferentially with the discovery of heteromers of receptors that are targets for addictive drugs or that are localized in brain circuits that are involved in addictive behaviors (such as dopamine, glutamate, cannabinoid, and adenosine receptors) and with the analysis of their biochemical and pharmacological properties involving studies at the cellular level as well as at the in vivo level.

Victor Fulgoni III, Ph.D., is currently senior vice president of Nutrition Impact, LLC, a consulting firm that helps food companies develop and communicate aggressive, science-based claims about their products and services. Nutrition Impact performs analyses of government food, nutrition, and health databases such as the National Health and Nutrition Examination Surveys for clients evaluating the contribution certain food and beverage products make to nutrient intake and their effect on certain health parameters. Dr. Fulgoni previously worked for the Kellogg Company as vice president of food and nutrition research, where he helped develop a long-term research program and was involved in the company's research and regulatory efforts to gain health claim approval from the FDA regarding soluble fiber from psyllium and the risk of heart disease.

Jeffrey Goldberger, M.D., a recognized scholar and clinician, has been a practicing clinical cardiac electrophysiologist at Northwestern University for 23 years. He is an innovator in the field and has been recognized as a "Top Doctor" by *U.S. News & World Report* and *Chicago* magazines. He has been a thought leader in the problems of sudden cardiac death, atrial fibrillation, and autonomic nervous system effects on cardiac electrophysiology, leading several multidisciplinary programs. He has written more than 200 publications, and he has served on multiple national committees of the American Heart Association and American College of Cardiology. Dr. Goldberger is an active participant in both undergraduate and graduate medical education and is involved in several community and national organizations in leadership roles.

Roland R. Griffiths, Ph.D., is professor in the Departments of Psychiatry and Neurosciences at the Johns Hopkins University School of Medicine. His principal research focus in both clinical and preclinical laboratories has been on the behavioral and subjective effects of mood-altering drugs. He is also a member of the Expert Advisory Panel on Drug Dependence for the World Health Organization (WHO). Dr. Griffiths's research has provided the most complete description of caffeine withdrawal syndrome to date, including documenting clinically significant functional impairment in some people. His research was the first to rigorously demonstrate the following: (1) that caffeine produces reliable mood-altering effects at doses far lower than previously thought possible; (2) that caffeine functions as a reliable reinforcer when administered in beverages or capsules; (3) that caffeine withdrawal potentiates the reinforcing effects of caffeine; and (4) that some people become psychiatrically dependent on caffeine in that they fulfill *Diagnostic and Statistical Manual* criteria for substance dependence applied to caffeine by being unable to quit despite repeated attempts to do so, by having a medical or psychological condition that is exacerbated by caffeine, and by continuing to use caffeine to avoid caffeine withdrawal symptoms.

John P. Higgins, M.D., M.B.A., is associate professor of medicine (cardiology) at the University of Texas Medical School, Houston, chief of cardiology at Lyndon B. Johnson General Hospital, and director of exercise physiology at the Institute for Sports Medicine and Human Performance at Memorial Hermann. Dr. Higgins was previously on the staff at the Veteran's Administration West Roxbury hospital as an attending cardiologist and director of the Cardiac Stress Laboratory (instructor in medicine, Harvard Medical School). He currently sees patients at Lyndon B. Johnson General Hospital. He has received the prestigious Dean's Teaching Excellence Award at the University of Texas Medical School at Houston 5 years in a row (2008–2013).

Diane C. Mitchell, M.S., R.D., is senior research scientist and the director of the Diet Assessment Center in the Department of Nutritional Sciences at the Pennsylvania State University. In this role she is responsible for managing external and internal research studies. She also manages proposal development, budget administration, manuscript development, and project management. Her research interests include validating and improving various diet assessment methodologies, accuracy and sources of error in diet recall, analysis of dietary patterns, diet quality, and database development. Ms. Mitchell is also scientific consultant to the International Life Science Institute of North America, Caffeine Working Group, to provide an update to earlier work on the caffeine intakes of the U.S. population.

Charles P. O'Brien, M.D., Ph.D., is the Kenneth E. Appel Professor of Psychiatry at the University of Pennsylvania. He also established and directs a clinical research program that has had a major impact on the treatment of addictive disorders. His work involves discovery of central nervous system changes involved in relapse, new medications, behavioral treatments, and instruments for measuring the severity of addictive disorders. He led the discovery of the effects of alcohol on the endogenous opioid system and developed a new treatment for alcoholism. Dr. O'Brien was elected to the Institute of Medicine (IOM) of the NAS in

1991, and he has received numerous research and teaching awards as well as an honorary doctorate from the University of Bordeaux. Dr. O'Brien is past president of the American College of Neuropsychopharmacology and the Association for Research in Nervous and Mental Disease. In 2013 the president of France named him Chevalier dans l'Ordre National de la Légion d'Honneur for his contributions to Franco-American scientific collaboration.

Ashley Roberts, Ph.D., is senior vice president in the Food and Nutrition Group at Intertek Cantox. In this capacity, Dr. Roberts advises and assists international clients with issues that are scientific, regulatory, and toxicological in nature. In addition, he assists clients wishing to design and develop scientific research programs and helps those who are developing regulatory strategies for food additives, foods that are generally recognized as safe, and novel foods. While in the food industry he was largely responsible for developing scientific strategies for establishing safety and gaining regulatory approvals for new food ingredients throughout the world. Prior to working for Intertek Cantox, Dr. Roberts worked in the area of scientific and regulatory affairs for a multinational food company for more than 10 years. Prior to that he worked in two leading European contract research organizations conducting drug metabolism and pharmacokinetics studies and phase I clinical trials.

Andrew P. Smith, Ph.D., is professor in the School of Psychology and director of the Centre for Occupational and Health Psychology at Cardiff University. His research covers the areas of occupational and health psychology with the major emphasis being on well-being. Specifically, Dr. Smith has conducted extensive research on the nonauditory effects of noise on cognition and health. In addition, he conducts research on stress and fatigue in both the workplace and life in general. Dr. Smith's interests in health psychology cover two main themes: health-related behaviors (effects of nutrition, caffeine, and chewing gum on behavior) and minor illnesses (psychosocial risk factors for susceptibility to colds and influenza; effects of upper respiratory tract infections on mood and cognition).

Jennifer Temple, Ph.D., is associate professor in the Departments of Exercise and Nutrition Sciences and Community Health and Health Behavior at the University of Buffalo. Dr. Temple is also director of the Nutrition and Health Research Laboratory in the School of Public Health and Health Professions at the University at Buffalo. Her research program focuses on several major areas, including physiological and behavioral effects of caffeine intake in children and adolescents, gender difference in the effects of caffeine, food reinforcement and sensory system influences on eating in adults, and the relationship between food reinforcement and weight change over time. Currently, Dr. Temple is investigating the cardiovascular, cognitive, subjective, and reinforcing effects of caffeine in pre- and post-pubertal children and across the menstrual cycle.

MODERATORS

Richard H. Adamson, Ph.D., is president of TPN Associates, LLC, a consulting firm specializing in toxicology, pharmacology, and nutrition issues. He spent 2 years as a commissioned officer in the U.S. Public Health Service and then became a civil servant at NIH. At NIH he was the director of the Division of Cancer Etiology and scientific director of the National Cancer Institute. In 1994 Dr. Adamson joined the American Beverage Association (ABA) as vice president for scientific and technical affairs. He retired from the ABA in December 2004. He has published more than 250 papers, serves on several editorial boards, and has received several honors and awards.

James R. Coughlin, Ph.D., is president of Coughlin & Associates. He has more than 35 years of experience in addressing and shaping the current understanding of food and nutrition science in the United States and Europe, particularly in the areas of food, chemical and environmental toxicology and safety, chemical risk assessment, risk-benefit evaluation of foods and food ingredients, generally recognized as safe (GRAS) food additive safety evaluations, and scientific risk communication. Before undertaking his current role as a consultant in 1991, he spent 10 years at General Foods Corporation and Kraft Foods Inc. managing external toxicology, safety, and regulatory affairs, including several years as Director of International Scientific Relations. Health and regulatory issues surrounding coffee/caffeine is one of his areas of expertise. In the early 1990s, he served as President of the Association for Science and Information on Coffee. He has been deeply involved in the assessment and management of California Proposition 65 requirements since the law's passage in 1986. He served for many years on the Editorial Advisory Board of Prop 65 News and the Prop 65 Clearinghouse Advisory Board.

Stephen R. Daniels, M.D., Ph.D., is professor of pediatrics and chairman in the Department of Pediatrics at the University of Colorado School of Medicine. He also serves as Pediatrician-in-Chief at Children's Hospital Colorado. Dr. Daniels's area of expertise is preventive cardiology, with a longtime interest in the application of sophisticated epidemiologic and biostatistical methods to pediatric clinical research problems. He is interested in the causes of blood pressure elevation and cholesterol abnormalities in children and adolescents, particularly the role that obesity may play in these health issues; development of structural and functional abnormalities in the heart and vascular system, including cardiovascular abnormalities occurring in pediatric patients with diabetes mellitus; as well as the relationship of left ventricular hypertrophy to obesity and hypertension. The role of lifestyle factors, such as diet and physical activity, is central to many of Dr. Daniels's studies.

Mark Feeley, M.Sc., is associate director of the Bureau of Chemical Safety in the Food Directorate of Health Canada. The Bureau of Chemical Safety of Health Canada is responsible for policy, standard setting, risk assessment, research, and evaluation activities with respect to chemicals in foods in Canada. Chemicals under the authority of the bureau include food additives; food packaging materials, processing aids, and incidental additives; food allergens; food contaminants; and novel foods. Mr. Feeley is the head of the Canadian delegation for the Codex Committee on Contaminants in Food, a current member of the Joint Food and Agriculture Organization/WHO Expert Committee on Food Additives Roster of Toxicological and Epidemiological Experts, and a member of the WHO Expert Advisory Panel on Food Safety.

Thomas J. Gould, Ph.D., is director of the Neuroscience Program, head of the Neurobiological Investigations of Learning & Addiction lab, and a professor of psychology at Temple University. In addition to affiliations with the psychology department and the neuroscience program, Dr. Gould has a secondary appointment in the Center for Substance Abuse Research at the Temple University School of Medicine, and he is also an investigator and member of the Center for Interdisciplinary Research on Nicotine Addiction at the University of Pennsylvania. His current research interest is the neurobiology of learning and memory with a specific focus on identifying the cellular and molecular events that underlie the effects of nicotine and ethanol on learning and memory. Current projects in the lab include an examination of the effects of nicotine on hippocampus functioning and hippocampus-dependent learning.

Steven E. Lipshultz, M.D., is chief of staff of Holtz Children's Hospital, Executive Associate Dean for Child Health, and Professor and Chairman of Pediatrics at the University of Miami, Miller School of Medicine. He has been the principal investigator in a number of groundbreaking NIH studies on the causes and treatment of cardiomyopathies in children. He studies the efficacy, long-term side effects, and outcomes of pharmacological agents in children using cross-sectional approaches. Another major focus of his research is development of surrogate outcome measures and biomarkers of adult-onset disease, such as coronary artery disease and health failure and prenatal and postnatal factors that moderate outcomes. Dr. Lipshultz has served on the faculties at Harvard Medical School and Boston University School of Medicine.

Barbara J. Petersen, Ph.D., M.P.H., is principal scientist in Exponent's Health Sciences Center for Chemical Regulation and Food Safety. She is also a specialist in addressing regulatory issues involving exposure and risk assessments including the FDA, the Environmental Protection Agency (EPA), and the European Food Safety Authority. Dr. Petersen chaired the WHO working group on methods for estimating intakes of food additives, nutrients, new biochemical traits associated with foods derived from modern biotechnology (genetically modified organisms), and contaminants in foods. She also served as Principal Investigator for the National Cancer Institute's International FOODBASE project, a major effort to collect and computerize descriptive and summary information on food consumption surveys conducted in more than 40 countries. Dr. Petersen has provided statistical support to the FDA's Center for Food Safety and Nutrition, including developing criteria for evaluating nutrition databases, and specifically for the International Interface Standard for food databases and to EPA's Office of Research and Development.

Joseph V. Rodricks, Ph.D., is a founding principal of ENVIRON, and an internationally recognized expert in toxicology and risk analysis. He has consulted for hundreds of manufacturers, government agencies and for the WHO in the evaluation of health risks associated with human exposure to chemical substances of all types. Dr. Rodricks came to consulting after a 15-year career as a scientist at the FDA. In his last 4 years at the FDA, he served as Associate Commissioner for Health Affairs. His experience extends from pharmaceuticals, medical devices, consumer products, and foods to occupational chemicals and environmental contaminants. He has served on the National Research Council's Board on Environmental Studies and Toxicology, and on 30 boards and committees of the NAS and the IOM.

Stephen Schaffer, Ph.D., is professor of pharmacology at the University of South Alabama. For 11 years, he served as a member of the American Heart Association Southeast Regional Consortium study section. His research interests include ischemia-reperfusion injury, the effects of diabetes and insulin on the heart, and the cardiac effects of the sulfur-containing amino acid taurine. Dr. Schaffer's work has been instrumental in establishing an important physiological role for taurine. In 1986 he discovered that taurine depletion caused a shift in energy metabolism of the heart in favor of glucose, an effect related to impaired mitochondrial function. He recently discovered that taurine deficiency leads to a decrease in the expression of mitochondria-encoded proteins, an effect that reduces the activity of the electron transport chain and enhances superoxide production by the mitochondria.

D

Workshop Statement of Task

An ad hoc committee will organize a 2-day public workshop to discuss potential health impacts stemming from the consumption of caffeine in dietary supplements and conventional foods, alone or in combination with other substances found in products commonly referred to as "energy products." The workshop will examine cardiovascular and central nervous system (CNS) effects and other important health hazards of caffeine that may arise in at-risk populations consuming varied amounts of caffeine. The committee will develop the agenda for the workshop, select and invite speakers and discussants, and moderate the discussions. The invited presentations and discussions will be structured to explore and discuss such topics as the following:

1. Evaluating the epidemiological, toxicological, clinical, and other relevant literature to identify and describe the important health hazards associated with caffeine and potential data gaps;
2. Delineating particular populations who may be at risk from caffeine exposure, taking into account interactive effects from other ingredients in "energy products" and preexisting medical conditions such as cardiovascular diseases;
3. Describing the risk for cardiovascular or other serious important health hazards for vulnerable populations, from exposure to caffeine-containing dietary supplements and conventional foods;
4. Identifying data gaps with regard to stimulant effects such as but not limited to caffeine on the cardiovascular and CNS systems; and
5. Exploring a safe level of exposure to caffeine for general and particular populations.

54